STOP BELLY-ACHING

STOP BELLY-ACHING

Banish Indigestion and Irritable Bowel Syndrome

Dr Peter Mansfield

Souvenir Press

This Edition published 2001 by
Souvenir Press Ltd.,
43 Great Russell Street, London WC13 3PD

Reprinted 2001, 2002

ISBN 0 285 63618 9

Typeset by Photoprint, Torquay, Devon
Printed in Great Britain

NOTICE TO READERS

Contents

page

Foreword   ix

Prelude

Chapter One: What is the Problem?   3

First Movement: Diet for Disaster

Chapter Two: Whatever did We do Before
                  Chemistry?   13
Chapter Three: The Evolution of Eating   22
Chapter Four: Our Waste of Taste   34
Chapter Five: Ration Roulette   47

Second Movement: Rationale for Recovery

Chapter Six: Read, Mark, Learn and Inwardly
                  Digest   71
Chapter Seven: Profoundly Moving   84

Third Movement: The Secrets of Success

Chapter Eight: The Natural Course of Events   105
Chapter Nine: An A-Z Guide to Food Choices   129

Chapter Ten: Special Diets   152
Chapter Eleven: Eating Out   165

Coda

Useful Addresses   173
Bibliography   178
Index   180

Foreword

The English language contains no phrase to match 'bon appetit!'. This says a lot about English-speaking people. We take too little care about what we eat and how we eat it. Mealtimes are becoming a thing of the past. Increasingly we snack in front of the TV or on the hoof. We eat in order to live, and take little pleasure in doing it.

This is by now so deeply ingrained that industry takes it for granted. Food is grown for quantity rather than quality, for cheapness rather than value, and for appearance rather than taste. It is processed for long-term storage and ease of preparation, pandering to our hectic lives. Even when we eat out, we are usually no better catered for.

As a result, quite a few of us cannot recall when last we ate a freshly prepared meal – let alone one using well grown ingredients. Many young people never have. Consequently, we have little or no conception of what we are missing.

What is worse, our knowledge of nutrition and digestive function is now entirely based on chemistry. Physical factors, such as the layout of our digestive organs or their mechanical behaviour are never considered – even by those we suppose to be experts. The impact of cooking methods, recipes and other culinary considerations gets only rudimentary attention. The partially sighted are leading the blind.

The digestive self-abuse that results has come to be known as Irritable Bowel Syndrome. All sorts of causes have been blamed for this epidemic since it emerged some decades ago. Some say it is based on allergy, some argue psychological disturbance, others blame stress. Any of these or all are capable of upsetting your tummy, certainly; but a robust tummy would not be so easily upset. No stomach can retain its native fortitude, however, in the face of the kind of abuse most of us hurl at it routinely, several times on every day of our lives – with extra helpings at our ritual feasts and on birthdays.

Thoughtful readers will wish to know why they have not heard this glaringly obvious message before, and what title I may have to expertise on the subject. I started my life as a promising student of the physical sciences but transferred to medicine in search of something more obviously of use to my fellow beings. This background made me look on medicine rather more broadly than most, and I gradually realised how narrowly most doctors think. After qualifying I discovered what health is, and radically rearranged my practice of medicine as a result. That brought home to me the key importance of what, when and how people eat. I traced and devoured all the wisdom I could find on the subject. It has been so utterly neglected recently that you might imagine its origins were prehistoric – yet most of it is less than a century old. I was eventually able to base most of my practice on the knowledge I acquired. In 1996 I gave up the struggle to do this as a NHS GP and concentrated on Good HealthKeeping (see Useful Addresses), the only serious attempt I know of to help its members keep out of the doctor's way.

Meanwhile I experiment continually on myself. From the beginning I radically altered my own diet, with benefits to my family and me that were quickly obvious. My wife and I began to take an interest in food and cuisine of all kinds, and we now eat very well at home and dine out regularly at good tables. Starting as bare necessity, it has become a hobby. I have planted the seed of similar success in many unlikely places. Yes: with all due modesty I think I may claim to know something of what I am talking about.

The rules for safe, satisfactory digestion and bowel function are very simple, and so are simply put. They are not always so simple to carry out, of course. The first impact of the right changes may feel catastrophic – sufficient to convince that you are making a great mistake. No, but decades of misuse have made your intestine flabby and lazy. When handled properly at last, its unpractised efforts are exaggerated, clumsy and uncomfortable. You need to reclaim it by gentle stages, just as you would any other organ you had forgotten you possess.

I am not so foolish as to suppose that this book will answer all your questions or solve all your problems. It should not, in any case, be taken as personal medical advice. I have written books before, and know better than to embark lightly on a new one. I feel deeply obliged, however, to resurrect this wide and powerful old perspective for you to explore, with or without professional assistance. Unless you know what I am about to tell you, bowel trouble will not only by irritable, but truly irresistible, and the best you can hope to do is stem the tide.

The purpose of this book runs deeper, however, than just to offer you real hope of a carefree, reliable and profoundly satisfactory digestion once more. This is only the first, but essential, step towards recovering all your profound capabilities. They are more stunted than you realise, for lack of grounding in the perfect digestion of good food. Reclaiming this is the beginning and seat of all real wisdom – of health, in fact. Health is nowadays in very short supply. To make it commonplace is the bottom line of everything I do.

Prelude

Chapter One: What is the problem?

I earn part of my living by ensuring the health of commercial pilots based in the East Midlands of the UK. Many of these pilots fly the helicopters that service the oil and gas rigs off the East coast. Their work is very demanding. They regularly have to cope with near gale-force winds howling across the small landing platforms of the rigs they visit. It is impossible to shut down the engines, as you normally would at an airport: the pilots have to carry on flying their machines even when on deck, to prevent them being blown away by a gust of wind.

Their visit to a rig is usually short, but each flight involves several hops from rig to rig before returning to base. Somewhere along the route a thoughtful chef will send up two parcels of sandwiches, one for each pilot. A basic skill such pilots learn, early in their careers, is to 'spell' each other while they take turns to get their sandwiches down.

Life on the rigs has its compensations, one of which is the standard of their catering. The sandwiches are thick slices of fresh bread generously filled with prawns or ham, mayonnaise or Thousand Islands dressing, watercress and lettuce – and very tasty too, I should imagine.

I learned all this some years ago from one of these pilots who was also a client of my NHS practice. He was attending for a routine repeat prescription for a modern, expensive, indigestion medicine. I have a rooted objection to this type of medicine because it prevents the formation of acid in the stomach which, as we shall see, is only required to digest rich protein food: a much cheaper way to achieve this is simply to avoid it. The pilot was not too receptive to this point at first, citing the difficult circumstances of his job in his defence.

So for several months we went on meeting like that, discussing the foul weather in the North Sea and mechanically repeating his prescription. But we made a little progress. He tried life without his tablets occasionally, and I got him to read one or two short leaflets in support of my contentions.

Eventually we hit upon the following experiment. Why not cherry-pick his sandwiches? He could try eating the fillings whilst he has a little time, hovering on deck; and save the bread and butter for later, in case he got hungry. He could probably manage to eat an empty sandwich during one of the longer hops, so long as he hadn't dropped it on the floor meanwhile.

At first this suggestion caused great mirth. What would his mates say? I told him to blame this crazy doctor, whom he was humouring. At least it would edge the weather out of the conversation occasionally.

I don't know when he first tried it. My oblique enquiries revealed very little for several months, during which his continued requests for prescriptions were not a good sign. Until one day when we met to renew his flying licence medical certificate, which is a different sort of encounter. When we got to examining his stomach he proudly announced that he had cured his indigestion. He had tried our plan intermittently at first, sometimes forgetting and sometimes just not bothering; but gradually it had become the rule rather than the exception. He found he did not always eat the bread at all, finding the crumpled, unsavoury package after the flight, inside his flying bag. We still meet every six months for aviation purposes but I am no longer his GP, so I cannot be sure what his consumption of medicines has been lately; but he is pleased with the money he is saving in prescription charges.

The trick responsible for the happy ending to this story will come home forcibly to you as we go through this book. It is so simple I wonder that in this instance it took the pilot and me so long to hit upon it. But that is the point, of course: we have become too thoroughly accustomed to expensive, high-tech fixes and cannot credit the understated, simple alternatives. It takes the mind of a child often to see the obvious, but most children of that age haven't yet got the facts to work on.

So let's look at the facts of bowel trouble. But first a few definitions, to save confusion. So far as this book is concerned, the 'gut' is a tube from mouth to anus. Most of it is the stomach followed by the small intestine, the main business part – referred to throughout the book simply as the 'intestine'. At the far end is a baggier part is the large intestine, or colon with all its attachments, referred to throughout as the 'bowel'. You will find all these terms illustrated and enlarged upon in the next chapter.

FALLING BETWEEN STOOLS

I have been a doctor long enough to see quite a few changes in the ways and extent to which people suffer. Chronic fatigue or post-viral syndrome has come from nowhere: hyperactivity and autism are no longer rare. The medical profession has, I fear, been late to recognise the reality and scale of problems such as these. Many members still don't. Medical investigations show no objective abnormalities in most sufferers of these complaints, and their symptoms are often not apparent when they attend the doctor's surgery. They are labelled as functional disturbances, often with an innuendo of mental or psycho-social origin, or even 'bad parenting'.

Irritable Bowel Syndrome is an exception. In some respects, medical observation and opinion have actually led the way. The reason for this sharp contrast lies in something called the index of suspicion. Doctors are trained to suspect dangerous conditions whenever symptoms appropriate to them appear, however common the symptoms and however rare the condition. In bowel cancer and inflammatory bowel conditions – such as Crohn's disease, coeliac disease and ulcerative colitis – the onset of abdominal pain or erratic bowel habit is an important clue, demanding further investigation. If no more serious cause is found, what is left is a normal intestine functioning abnormally: an irritable bowel. In the absence of positive tests, the diagnosis is based entirely on symptoms, and in the jargon of medicine a collection of symptoms is called a syndrome. Irritable Bowel Syndrome (IBS for short) is therefore more logically named than most medical conditions.

Serious attention in the scientific journals began in 1962 and the foundations of the modern definition were laid in 1978. The key references up to date are listed at the end of this chapter.

They generally agree that around 15–20 per cent of the population, mostly adult and female, now have at least four of the typical symptoms at any one time. The symptoms on which the diagnosis is based are: distension; abdominal pain relieved by emptying the bowel; change in frequency, consistency, ease of passage or completeness of emptying of bowel motions; and the presence of mucus in them. Only a fifth of sufferers consult their doctors, and from those that do are drawn 30–50 per cent of all referrals to specialist intestinal clinics in hospitals. Nobody knows the root cause of the condition, though its main features have been established and some precipitating causes have been identified. Treatment in general has not, until now, been very successful. There is certainly no 'magic bullet' prescription that works in all cases.

The bowel irritability has two aspects: strong, easily provoked, erratic contractions of the bowel muscle on the one hand, and greater sensitivity to pain from distension on the other. The question is what causes them. For once, genes and heredity do not seem to be much involved. IBS starts as an after-effect in 24–37 per cent of cases of acute bowel infection, but this accounts for only a small minority of all cases of IBS. A diet containing too little vegetable fibre is suspect, but treating the condition with fibre substitutes does not work. This finding is weakened by the fact that treatment is usually with doses of bran from cereals, which is often contaminated with pesticides sprayed on the crop before harvest (see Chapter Five): none of the studies took this into account. It is an important oversight because nearly half of all IBS sufferers improve dramatically when foods they cannot tolerate are removed from their diets. Pesticide intolerance is an important potential cause of many irritation symptoms. Pesticides are fat-soluble, and even pure fatty acids or bile acids that reach the bowel usually provoke symptoms in IBS patients. However half of IBS cases with food intolerance (25 per cent of the total) involve carbohydrates or complex sugars, commonly lactose from milk.

That still leaves around half of all IBS cases unaccounted for, however. A few cases turn out to be the direct result of chronic infection with abnormal germs in the bowel, usually as a result of prolonged antibiotic treatment. Some have a clear relation to emotional factors or other life stresses, and it would be easy to dump all remaining cases on subtler expressions of that cause. This does not, however, explain why some people under pressure produce bowel symptoms instead of, for example, headaches or chest pain.

Very few of the medical texts I have seen on the subject discuss the possible relationship of IBS to other gut disorders. This is chiefly because of the strong tendency for medical specialists to distinguish everything by putting them into separate compartments. We do not even know whether or not children with tummy-ache become adults with IBS. However, IBS does seem to overlap other intestinal disturbances such as indigestion.

Does IBS ever herald worse disease to come? It never coincides with them of course, by definition; but it could be the foothills from which mountains spring. Coeliac disease, a strong intolerance of wheat gluten, is an extreme example of the slower, lower-grade intolerances that explain about half of IBS; so there's one mountain, anyway. Diverticular disease is part and parcel of prolonged chronic constipation, for reasons discussed in Chapter Seven. A chronically overactive bowel is much more likely than a normal one to produce diverticula, making that a particularly high foothill, if not a separate mountain.

When an attack of ulcerative colitis subsides, IBS may persist. Nobody has commented on the reverse situation, however, of ulcerative colitis eventually superseding previous IBS. Neither condition has a known cause. Genes contribute little or nothing to either. It does seem possible that ulcerative colitis represents an extreme form of gut irritability, affecting relatively few especially susceptible people. Much the same factors that provoke ulcerative colitis in the vulnerable few are getting to more people now. Perhaps they have intensified, or perhaps new forms of irritation have come into effect. Either way, they have produced a rapid increase of IBS in a wider population who used not to be susceptible. The ulcerative colitis mountain was always there: the IBS foothills around it have risen up and spread out in recent decades.

Crohn's disease is rather distinct. Its main features are quite different from ulcerative colitis. It affects more of the gut, whereas ulcerative colitis is confined to the bowel and chiefly its far end. It is three times commoner in smokers, whereas ulcerative colitis is precisely the opposite. It suddenly became twice to three times as common in England and Wales during the 1960s, and may now be declining again; whereas ulcerative colitis has not increased recently and is rather more common anyway. Genetic predisposition is much more significant in Crohn's disease. However, environmental factors, such as high sugar and low vegetable fibre intake, still play a large part. Attempts to correct the disease by restoring the fibre and reducing sugar have failed, perhaps for the reason already suggested for IBS – contamination of the fibre with irritant pesticides. However a gut with Crohn's disease heals up when no food at all passes through it, which indicates that food is in some way deeply involved. So Crohn's disease is a contrasting mountain, with unique geology, that may have been nudged upwards a little as the foothills spread.

Cancer of the bowel has some dietary causes in common with IBS, in particular low fibre intake and perhaps intake of animal fats. It is definitely more common in ulcerative colitis, developing in 5–10 per cent of cases after 20 years of widespread disease. Cancer of the intestine is more common after prolonged Crohn's disease, but much rarer anyway than cancer of the bowel. Cancer in the intestine, or indeed in any part of the gut, is more common in people with coeliac disease. So cancer represents the snow-line that never leaves the mountains, and in bad weather reaches the hills more easily, only reaching the valley below in the most extreme conditions.

Where do all these fragments of information get us? Obviously the science of this subject is full of holes, and the field is wide open for bright ideas. I think the explanation of all these conditions is fundamentally the same, is in principle very simple, but runs very deep. It is set out in detail in the next part of this book.

Digestive self-abuse was always sufficient to provoke ulcerative colitis, Crohn's disease and Coeliac disease in contrasting groups of particularly susceptible people, and IBS symptoms occur alongside other features in all of them. The rising tide of gut abuse has, however, forced increasing numbers of normal people beyond their powers of resistance into the same symptom pattern. And if your gut's capacity to cope is breached, and never allowed to recover, bowel cancer is the eventual risk, regardless of your starting point.

So IBS is a wake-up call to everyone. It's time to right a great, insidious wrong we are allowing to overwhelm us gradually. This will also restore one of our most vivid pleasures, so you won't lack motivation once you've made a start. Read on.

First Movement
Diet for Disaster

Chapter Two: Whatever did We do Before Chemistry?

It takes ten years to turn a reasonably bright student into a doctor incapable of thinking straight. Our modern preoccupation with chemistry has completely obscured many elementary principles about our bodily functions that were crystal clear to far more people – including some doctors – a century ago.

It was very vivid to me. I went up to Cambridge in 1962, less than ten years after the structure of DNA had been identified there by Crick and Watson. Biochemistry was by then the most glamorous subject you could study, staffed with young raunchy dons in command of unbelievable research funds and book advances. The subject was developing so fast that, as part of your revision for each year's exams, you needed to attend the latest course of lectures all over again – so radically had all the theories changed from one year to the next. Many of my contemporaries took up research and teaching posts in younger universities, which were just opening departments of biochemistry run by some of the youngest professors ever.

It was later that the historical significance of all this dawned on me. The departments of chemistry had also been doing very nicely at that time. Where were the billions, required for these massive institutions to stay open, coming from? Not from student fees of course, but industry. Some students were being funded through their studies by industrial sponsors, but the big money was going directly into the teaching and research departments. The motive is obvious – to develop new, value-added chemical products, especially for applications in agriculture and medicine.

This still doesn't quite explain the huge energy being devoted to it, just at that time. But parallels from agriculture make me think that it was a consequence of the huge increase in primary chemical production sparked off by the Second World War. Something similar happened during the Great War, but because global transport was still quite limited in scale it did not achieve the turnover that was to arise during the early 1940s. And of course, the aftermath of the Great War was grossly mismanaged. The shipbuilding, automotive and munitions industries were simply allowed to slump, carrying the entire economy with them.

Someone in the 1940s, I know not who, had the sense to manage things differently. Thank goodness they did, or the mother of all slumps would have overtaken us then. Instead, they set about finding peacetime uses for all the heavy machinery factories and chemical raw materials. This, I am convinced, was behind the drive to use chemical fertilisers more widely in agriculture – the nitrates on which fertilisers are based happen also to be a major ingredient of many explosives! To persuade farmers to use them, and teach them how, we needed chemistry graduates. For chemistry graduates we needed larger university departments of chemistry.

It did not all end there, of course. The best minds in chemistry were set to work, in the same universities, on research grants to find more sophisticated applications for the raw materials that were in such plentiful supply. Pharmaceuticals were virtually unknown before 1940, and penicillin was brand new – what potential! Pharmaceutical shares soared, and they remain blue chips to this day.

The key to that was a combination of patent law and bio-chemistry. Industry needed to find new chemical entities that would do useful things in the human body, so we needed to know how the chemistry of the body worked – hence the departments of biochemistry. Patent law, meanwhile, was the key to billion-pound profits. Whoever discovered a particular new chemical first could patent it and be immune from competition for the first 16 years of its exploitation. If the chemical proved really useful, they could name their price. If the use was pharmaceutical they had to get a product licence for it first, which takes a large part of the patent period – so the winners probably only have about five years to get back their outlay. Consequently the market price they set can be astronomical. This keeps the research laboratories funded, in the universities and now in the larger companies, and the cycle sustains itself.

Meanwhile it was also necessary to get doctors around to the chemical way of thinking. So industrial funds started flowing into medical laboratories too, and on into medical schools. Large numbers of graduates (not all chemists) were recruited by drug houses to represent their interests to doctors in their practices. Most GPs faced dozens of requests for appointments with drug reps every month. This quickly became tedious for them, so more and more subtle inducements were employed to get the GPs' attention – lunch with a message, toys for the desk, trips to medical conferences that just happened to be in exotic places – all easily affordable by companies out of the profits on their current drug patents. This below-the-belt marketing grew a little out of hand and guidelines for good practice are now in force, but the inputs are still there through funding for post-graduate medical institutes and other laudable ventures. No wonder most doctors behave as if there were a pill for every ill!

I used to see a few of these reps and remember the occasion on which I realised how hollow all this is. I interrupted one with a question, a few minutes into his piece. He dealt with this and tried to resume his message, obviously thrown. In the end he said, 'I'm afraid I've lost the thread – d'you mind if I start again?' – and began once more, word perfect. He had learned the whole thing by rote, like an actor's lines. I terminated the ridiculous charade, gave him coffee and we had a chat instead.

And that, I believe, is how it came about that we forgot – in less than fifty years – the other 95 per cent of what health is about. The drive for chemistry may have been justified to keep the show on the road after the war, or we should never have 'had it so good'. But it has become a life-threatening bandwagon, and nobody seems to know how to get off. The global pharmaceutical giants are now far more powerful than governments or even international economic communities, not least because they think decades ahead – politicians manage no more than a few years. Senior politicians understand the need to modify patent law as it applies to medicines, but feel powerless to do so. We cannot wait for the powers-that-be in pharmaceuticals to wake up to the situation. We must wake up ourselves.

BURIED TREASURE

Doctors who question this situation drift into the hands of devotees, and that is what happened to me. I joined an outfit called the McCarrison Society whose primary concern was to keep alive a sense of the importance of properly grown food for human health. In the 1960s that was not a common attitude; that most people now at least pay lip-service to it is a measure of their success. Most of its members were grand people whom I feel privileged to have known. They introduced me to a stock of old books, long out of print, expressing even older ideas that set my pulse racing.

Throughout the nineteenth century and well into the last, there was a huge preoccupation with health that was far more intelligent than anything we have now. Some of it was faddist, but most of it hammered home essentially the same message – that we are what we eat, breathe, drink, think and do. But it went further, noting curious observations about the different effects of food and drink that had been grown and prepared in different ways. A brilliantly clear definition of health was available by 1945, taking full account of all this, which we have yet to make anything of. And the chief reason for this? – nobody can make any real money out of it.

This view may sound jaded and cynical, but you have only to measure it against some of the perplexing opinions we get from our doctors, industrialists and politicians to realise that it makes far too much sense. There is no profit for the chemical industry in simple remedies, wholesome food or healthy people – it is as simple as that.

But let us not be side-tracked. We need to meet some of the great characters who wrote these old books, many of whom led exceedingly vivid and interesting lives. In any case, their insights will crop up in some detail in later chapters, and this is an appropriate point to introduce them.

My enlightenment began with Robert McCarrison, as I said. He was a doctor and lieutenant colonel in the Indian Medical Service at the time of the Great War, and made some astute observations of the diverse tribal populations of India and their habits of living. He went on to demonstrate a direct link between their customary food and disease patterns by feeding well kept pigeons and rats in similar ways. His experiments differed from most modern feeding experiments in that he only selected the kind of food the animals had available, to correspond with the diet of the tribal group in question, and left the animal to balance it according to its appetite. His work was praised by many of his peers as the best of its kind in the world at the time.

One of those peers was Arbuthnot Lane, a surgeon in the UK who became celebrated for his work on diseases of the colon. Gross, long-established constipation was rife at the time, for reasons we shall see later. He frequently felt called upon to remove the entire colon in order to cure his patient, so far beyond repair did he find it. The effects were often remarkable and led some contemporary surgeons to advocate removal of the colon as routine preventive medicine – which would by coincidence be highly profitable to them. Lane did not agree; but he deduced why the colon was so often drastically degenerate, and what its normal function was.

The only book of his that I possess does not deal with this accomplishment, which I read about in another by Are Waerland, a Swedish doctor who spent much of his life in England and wrote quite masterfully in his adopted language. He told the story of hygiene from the Middle Ages in such an engaging way I could hardly put it down. Referring to Lane and another contemporary, Ellis Barker, he makes it obvious that diseases most often cause germs, rather than the other way round – a view expounded in more detail by Antoine Béchamp, a contemporary of Pasteur – and that the composition of germs in the bowel is a key to health. It is interesting how clearly this presents itself to him, with a fraction of the bacteriological knowledge that we now possess – an example of the truth becoming lost in a vast white noise of mere information. Nobody nowadays has anywhere near his insight, which I will share with you in due course.

Max Bircher-Benner is senior to them all historically, though his writings and insights feel much more recent. He founded a world-famous nature-cure clinic in Zurich which bore his name. He also invented muesli, to which modern cereal products of that name bear only a very distant resemblance. He is, so far as

I know, the physician who first made practical and brilliant use of the distinction between live and dead food.

He in turn made use of even earlier work by Father Sebastian Kneipp, a nineteenth-century priest in the parish of Bad Wörishofen in Bavaria. Of necessity, he had been the principal agent of healing in his remote part of the world, with only the wild forces of nature to help him. He devised the basis of hydrotherapy, or water-cure, as it is still practised today and taught in the eponymous Institute in his home town. This is not, by the way, the mere use of a swimming pool to bear the weight of patients regaining the use of their limbs – far from it. You will learn more about that when we need to introduce a few of the details, later on.

That is backwards far enough. We return to the last century to meet another group of contributors to my enlightenment. The one to whom I am most drawn is Dr Lionel Picton, a medical officer of health in Cheshire around 1940. His career bears considerable resemblance to my own – a general practitioner, with part-time public responsibilities and a flair for concerted action. There the resemblance ends, because his powers of observation and deduction were very acute and illuminating, and his activities more successful. I attribute especially to him the realisation that in practice we humans have two stomachs. There is no misprint: you understand me correctly.

An approximate contemporary of his was Arnold Ehret, an emigré professor of music in North America. He developed chronic nephritis, a life-threatening inflammatory disease of the kidneys. This entailed losing huge amounts of protein through his urine, which his physicians struggled to replace in his diet. This made matters worse, and it seemed sensible to Ehret to try the opposite approach. He did this without the knowledge and to the eventual embarrassment of his doctors – because within two years he was completely cured. This led him to visualise excess protein in the body as constituting a sort of internal mucus, which causes chronic disease by generally getting in the way and souring everything – very much in line with Lane and Waerland, whom he probably did not know about. He devised his mucus-less diet to deal with the problem, and I still regard this – despite its quaint name – as the best all-round curative diet available. Ehret's work was recognised by Benedict Lust, a pioneer of naturopathy and perhaps the originator of that term. Lust published Ehret's dietary recommendations as a series of pamphlets, which may still be in print.

America at that time was alive with interest in health and natural methods of treatment. Two particular individuals deserve mention – Weston Price and Francis Pottenger. Price was a distinguished dentist whose great legacy was a monumental anthropological survey comparing the effects of traditional and modern diets on the teeth and jaws of a wide variety of national and tribal groups. It is hard to imagine how anything remotely as good would ever be accomplished now by an entire expedition, let alone one man.

Pottenger was a physician, like his father, and at one point conducted research using cats. He had considerable trouble with deaths among his cat breeding stock and changed the direction of his research to find out why. His cat feeding experiments demonstrated the disastrous effects on these carnivores of cooking their meat or milk, such that they were unable to rear healthy young within eighteen months of starting on cooked food. Once their diet was restored, it took up to five years to regain their health, and never did they regain their ability to rear well favoured young. Unfortunately for us humans, precisely similar effects were obvious in children he later examined, with weakening of the hormonal and physical contrast between boys and girls. Osteoporosis, as well as sexual ambiguity, was firmly established by Pottenger to be a consequence of pasteurisation of milk and lack of raw food generally.

A curious extension of his work was revealed when the pens in which his cats had lived were sown with beans. The plants in the raw food cages were far more verdant and productive than those in the pens fertilised with urine and faeces from animals fed only cooked food. It seems that the modern emphasis in public hygiene on bacteriological sterility is a profound mistake, the ramifications of which we shall be exploring.

Next comes Surgeon Captain T.L. Cleave – I never discovered his first names – who in the 1960s wrote an illuminating account of his escapades as a naval surgeon. Picture only the many sacks of bran that were always taken on a ship he was in, and imagine the parades on board at which spoonsful of it were administered to reluctant sailors under his watchful eye, and you have some impression of the man. His gift was to discern the extent of the diseases caused by sugar consumption. He actually thought of them as one seamless condition: the saccharine disease.

I come next to Doris Grant, and through her to William Howard Hay. Doris is the only one of these people whom I have known personally and corresponded with. My wife and I had been baking wholemeal bread to her recipe for years, without knowing its creator. She subsequently wrote with Jean Joice an exposition of Hay's work, which became a huge best-seller.

Hay was an American physician who, like Ehret, learned about disease largely by curing himself. He lived in a society very fond of its meat. Every member of it had something approaching a patriotic duty to consume at least one T-bone steak a day. This was responsible for a great deal of toxic illness which Hay understood and defused, largely by identifying the importance of separating into different meals foods that require different types of digestion. Actually, the French had unconsciously beaten him to it and gone one up on him, but they did not have to contend with quite such voracious beef-eaters. We shall explore the details of food combining at the proper time.

The last of my gurus is also the youngest, Michel Montignac. As representative in Paris of a major multinational company, he was obliged to entertain many visitors to the best his country has to offer. High on the list was French food, which was putting weight on Michel at an alarming rate. He went into his firm's database to find out what to do about this, and discovered how way off beam most weight reduction diets are. He proved the success of his researches before writing his first book *Eat Yourself Slim*, which met with international success. We are not here primarily concerned with weight control, but Montiguac's insights revealed the last piece of the jigsaw of bowel behaviour.

SPUN HERITAGE

That's quite a line-up. And they form a minority of the examples available, who happen to have contributed directly to the subject matter of this book. You may have heard of muesli, but had you any idea otherwise that any of these people ever existed? If not, pause to reflect on the awesome speed with which important lessons are forgotten these days – in the so-called information age. Our prehistoric ancestors did better by telling stories round their camp fires. Our own times are really, and less honourably, the age of information management. We are far too good at burying knowledge we find inconvenient or unprofitable.

This meteoric transition – from the age of health to that of chemistry in about thirty years – might have been justified if everything about health could be explained in terms of chemistry: but it cannot. Chemistry gives an account of what elements exist in a cabbage or a courgette, how they are combined into molecules, and how those molecules interact with each other in the daily life of the plant. It gets nowhere near explaining how this complex array of biochemicals becomes structured in any consistent form, let alone that of a specific vegetable plant species. Biologists are, unfortunately and with precious few exceptions, no better placed. They can describe, compare and contrast plant and animal structures and speculate about their evolution, but they cannot account for the growth and development of form in any of them.

To allow our biological heritage and potential to be so completely usurped by a half-science sponsored by commercial interest was a monstrous folly, which must eventually be redeemed. We begin that process by opening our eyes to it personally, and to its disastrous effects in ourselves. Successful repair of those effects by relieving their causes – mercifully still possible, with time, for most of us – will testify to the utility and truth in what I have said so far.

But first we must spell out in more detail what would by now be common knowledge, had not the business perspective taken so large a hand.

References
Representative titles are listed in the bibliography to justify what I have said, and for readers to explore more deeply if they wish. Most of them are, unfortunately, long out of print and unobtainable through the library system, but antiquarian book dealers are often able to trace second hand copies to private commission. The Wholefood Bookshop, 24 Paddington Street, London W1 stocks some titles from time to time, as they become available.

Chapter Three: The Evolution of Eating

PALAEO-ARROGANCE

We talk rather glibly of evolution these days, as if it were all cut and dried. Actually, there are many riddles concerning the way in which the living creatures of this earth have evolved, none of which is yet solved by the science we have signed up to on the subject. Any suggestion that we yet know it all is arrogant in the extreme.

The largest puzzle does not concern us directly, but illustrates the scale of our presumption in theorising about evolution at all – let alone with confidence. Everything starts with the fossil record, the only hard data we can possibly have about prehistoric times. What that record seems to suggest is that not one but several attempts have been made on earth to evolve a successful population of living things. Each attempt started higher (on an arbitrary evolutionary scale with humans at the top, of course) and moved forward a little further than the previous one, came to a full flowering of refinement, and then disappeared completely. This has happened several times, according to the palaeontological record. The so-called age of the dinosaurs is only the best known of these epochs.

So what have we made of this?

Our modern assumption is that we simply haven't yet found the links in between that would make it a continuous record of the smooth ascent of *Homo sapiens*. That is the most comfortable fit with Darwin's proposed survival of the fittest, and with modern genetic interpretations of that theory; but it is not being borne out by any new fossil discoveries.

However, the existing record could be interpreted otherwise. Maybe there truly have been several separate waves of evolution, each one like a drawing somebody has begun, been dissatisfied with, and scrapped before starting again. That deals neatly with the way each epoch starts off better than the last, but suggests divine intervention of some kind too strongly for modern tastes – one hardly dare mention it out loud. More palatable is the idea that evolution has, indeed, started several times but failed each time to adapt sufficiently to the evolving geography of the earth, and has perished for that reason. Why, then, does the next evolutionary epoch always seem to contain the memory of the previous ones? And does that suggest the emergence of life was somehow inevitable or deliberate, rather than a convenient but accidental collision of the right molecules at some time?

I offer no answers for any of these questions. Clearly fitter species do survive better than ill adapted ones. The issue is whether that is the only available mechanism for evolution, and whether it accounts adequately for the depth of intelligence we see in nature today. I suspect not. For the moment, however, I wish only to establish the legitimacy of speculating about human evolution along unconventional lines. If there are major doubts about the parts of animals that are hard and fast enough to survive in fossil form, how much more reasonable still to muse liberally about the softer part – such as intestines. And that is precisely what I now intend to do.

FRUITS OF EDEN

Whatever may have been our ancient prehistory, our present concerns begin with the first human creatures of the current evolutionary epoch. They arrive on the scene anywhere between 40 million and 2 million years ago – the precise timing does not much affect our line of reasoning. Whenever human creatures began, most plant and many animal species had preceded them by tens or hundreds of millions of years.

It seems certain that the tropical rain forest was already widely established and richly populated with a huge diversity of creatures, all living without difficulty on the abundant fruits and shoots of the forest, if not upon each other. Despite everything that has happened since – however much the primaeval forest may be in retreat in the face of latterday industrial development

– it still seems to represent faithfully our most ancient environmental heritage.

From what we can tell, the earliest human creatures made their homes there or thereabouts. Food in the forest has never presented a problem – you have only to reach for it as you force your way through the thicket. Live, raw, tender shoots, fruit or nuts are there to be had at any time of year. We know from the experience of modern vegans that it is possible to sustain a long life on food confined to these sources, though you do not easily get fat on it. Leanness stands out as unusual in this century, when our relative idleness uses little energy and we grow obese too easily.

Our earliest ancestors worked much harder physically, of course, and needed lots of energy-giving food to keep going. Nuts and seeds would therefore have been at a premium, being both richly endowed with energy (to sustain the seed during germination, before it starts feeding from the soil) and relatively scarce. Most fruits, however abundant, yield far less energy interspersed with lots of moisture and fibrous material. Biologically they seem set out to be attractive rather than sustaining, so that animals will swallow the seeds they contain and disperse them to sprout and take root elsewhere, away from the parent plant. To get enough energy from this, the most readily available food, primitive humans had therefore to eat huge amounts of it.

They were probably eating pretty well all day long, very much like grazing animals still do. The similarity between the intestines of modern humans, and grazing or herbivorous animals, strongly corroborates this. Our present much smaller reliance on vegetation would never have called into being such elaborate guts, however they were evolved. We must, even in the relatively recent past, have eaten much more plant matter than we do now. This is therefore our most primitive food and our intestines are well adapted to dealing with it. Fresh raw leaves, fruit or shoots entering the intestine are recognised and welcomed comfortably as entirely familiar by the skin lining it. These remain, even now, our best foods for convalescence after any kind of digestive upset – as we shall see.

This huge reliance on vegetation by primitive humans has a number of ramifications we should take note of at this stage, because of their significance today.

WASTE DISPOSAL

To get the kind of energy they needed, primitive forest people would have eaten their way through the equivalent of about 40 modern apples or 30 bananas a day. These descendants of the original fruits would also yield respectively 12 or 36 grams of protein, 4½ or 2½ litres of water and 44 or 18 grams of indigestible fibrous material. We can be reasonably sure that ancient wild varieties would have had less water and lots more fibre: let's assume the protein content per unit of energy yield was about the same. That means our most primitive ancestors got by on less than 45 grams of protein daily – which is very close to what experts say we need now.

We seem to be thinking along the right lines, so let's look where else they lead. The weight of modern fruit the ancestors would have had to eat for these results is colossal – between 3½ and 5½ kilograms, or up to 12 pounds! But the ancient counterparts would have been less massive and watery, so let's suppose they were eating more like 3 kilograms every day. That would have contained around 2 litres of water, so they probably didn't get thirsty or drink much else – which is perhaps just as well, since they were also excreting rather freely, and contaminating nearby water sources. If we assume that they had to deal with around 100 grams of undigested fibre each day, their bowels would have cleared about 250 grams of faeces or nearly four times the typical modern amount. That's quite possible – African tribes today subsisting mostly on maize go 50 per cent higher than that. But it means at least three bowel clearances each day – in modern terms, a motion after every meal.

Whilst there is nothing in this mass production line to indicate how fast a meal would progress from stem to stern through the intestine, we can assume transit only took a matter of hours. Otherwise the weight of our ancestors' guts would have rivalled the average cow's, and we'd never have made it on to our feet. What's more, the journey through most of it – now called the small intestine, about 10 metres long – must have been very quick, to avoid bloating. Most of those few hours would have been spent in the predecessor of the modern large intestine, or bowel, which is of much larger diameter and about two metres long.

The evolutionary separation of intestine and bowel is a classic chicken and egg situation: which came first? It seems very improbable that our ancestors ever managed without some sort of reservoir at the end of their guts, to stop them having to leak a trail of tell-tale faeces all the time. Without that, our unfortunate forest-dwellers would have been squatting every few minutes, literally sitting targets for the many man-eating animals they shared the forests with and a clear candidate for extinction of the unfit. Then again, we must have been making much better use of the bowel in the remote past than we have since Victorian times, or Arbuthnot Lane and his contemporaries would not have been called on to remove so many of them surgically.

AFTER-BURNER

We begin to see where some of our current problems lie, and they are not just a question of throughput. Climate change has not only been global, but intestinal too.

The cellulose fibre component of a primitive human diet is very succulent – there's no need to chew woody old shoots with so many fresh buds and fruits to choose from. Locked into the architecture of this fibre is quite a lot of moisture and some starches, that would have been accessible but for the cellulose barrier. As always in nature, where there's food of any kind there's also something ready to eat it. In this case, germs capable of digesting cellulose live on the plant's surface, and get eaten along with it.

They don't have time to get to work in the torrential flow through the intestine, but can multiply in the relative calm of the bowel beyond. Some of the cellulose is therefore split open, letting out the starches within. These in turn nourish a wider variety of other germs that have been consumed along with the meal, as well as the cellulose-splitters. So a considerable colony of germs can be maintained in the bowel, as long as its owner continues to eat plenty of fresh cellulose regularly. This colony is self-sustaining: you do not need to reinforce it constantly with new germs from outside. However, later additions to our food would have brought with them new immigrant germs – some of which settled very well into this scenario, as we shall see (p. 150).

Because all these germs were taking advantage of cellulose and the starches they contain, the end-products of their digestive processes would have been the innocuous acids of various kinds that arise naturally from breakdown of these substances. To survive this fouling of their own nest, the germs had to be comfortable in acid conditions. In the terminology of biologists, Greek to the rest of us, these acid-loving germs are labelled *acidophilus*.

This means that we evolved with an acidic climate in the bowel, and learned to take advantage of it. Huge colonies of acid-forming bacteria conducted a secondary digestion of the vegetable remains of each meal, creating the 'vitamins' they needed in their own bodies and surrendering them to us when they died. This is how vegans in all ages have managed to get enough vitamin B12, for example, which chiefly occurs in meat foods: the germs in their bowels made the vitamin for them.

EXCESS BAGGAGE

We can extend this fruitful line of reasoning in other ways. Linus Pauling drew attention to the large amount of Vitamin C our ancestors would have eaten on an exclusively vegetable and fruit diet. I am not now convinced with the force of all his arguments, but it seems clear that rain forest humans would have consumed at least several times the amount of every vitamin they required each day, along with the energy they needed.

Vitamins are 'vital' because we cannot make them for ourselves, and because of the vital functions they support. Without them we cannot get at the energy we eat, for example, and turn it into a useful form. In nature, most creatures only abandon the apparatus for making something vital when it is so abundant in their surroundings that they never run short of it. In those circumstances, the unnecessary apparatus becomes an encumbrance that slows the organism down. Imagine the performance of a racing car that carried its own fuel refinery.

We humans have long ago stopped making vital food components we have always been able to rely on. We cannot re-acquire the ability to make vitamins so easily as we lost it, so we are forced to ensure that we always eat enough. We shall come to the implications of this in Part Two.

MOVING ON

However, there are problems living in the tropics and a large human population could never be at home there. Even today, primitive tribes-people in the rain forest mostly die of falls, snake-bite or mauling by big cats. So quite early on our ancestors moved away from the forests, first to the lakes and riversides and eventually to the sea coast. Gradually they moved away from the tropics into what are called temperate latitudes. The dangers are fewer here, but the seasons become more important. Shoots and fruit tend not to be available in winter and will not keep right through from the autumn. So to cope with this our ancestors had to learn to hunt and fish, and then to digest what they had caught.

That requires a careful balancing act. Animal flesh is similar to human, so the process for digesting meat can also digest intestines. That mistake happens regularly today and results in gastritis and ulcers. To cope, we developed a stomach at the beginning of the intestine which can make the acid juices required to break down meat, but also makes sufficient mucus to hold the stomach's contents away from its lining and prevent the acid from burning holes in it. Such an adaptation must have been completed several million years ago, but much more recently than any division of intestine from bowel. A bulky vegetable diet creates an urgent need for a bowel, as we have seen; but until we started to eat flesh we would not have needed a stomach at all.

One other 'invention' was necessary to enable the human intestine, which is chiefly designed for food from plants, to deal also with meat. Carnivorous animals have short intestines – if they yawn you can practically see right through – because live meat ferments quickly and rotten meat would make the animal very ill if retained more than an hour or two. We overcome this threat not by shortening our intestines but by cooking the meat before we eat it. This slows down fermentation so that it has hardly got underway before we have expelled the remains, six to twelve hours later.

Successful hunting, fishing and meat-eating enabled human populations to subsist throughout the year almost anywhere on earth. Mastery of meat and of iron presumably developed alongside each other, because both required using fire constructively – itself a considerable step forward. And of course the ability to fashion iron tools greatly increased the efficiency of hunting, and in due course cooking too. So, as archaeology goes, this whole trend would have been explosively fast.

The very speed of it means it can never have been entirely comfortable. Some meals would go down well, others badly. Whenever a decent kill was made, the entire clan would have to gorge on it before rot set in, probably then resting for a day or so to let the huge meal digest. In time they developed ways of prolonging its life in storage, though never quite preserving it in the modern sense. Even the efficiently smoked meats and fish we can buy now cannot be kept for long without deep refrigeration.

Any foul meat eaten, or slow-down in the transit of even fresh meat through the intestine – what we would now call constipation – encourages meat fermentation despite the cooking. This produces a hostile bowel climate against which the bowel lining reacts irritably. This irritation takes the form of inflammation, the basic recovery mode of all the body's tissues. It can be provoked by infection, but usually isn't. The modern assumption that gastro-enteritis is caused by a germ or its toxin is seldom correct. As a matter of fact, germs more often take advantage of and multiply in a tissue that is already weakened or inflamed, than cause that inflammation in the first place. It is important to appreciate this fundamental point, which we shall return to repeatedly later.

Tummy upsets and gastro-enteritis are names we give to short-term irritation of this kind. Trouble has become chronic – indeed epidemic – in recent times, because the causes of irritation have multiplied and never go away. Some people have never experienced anything else. Chronic irritations go deeper and get more stubborn with time. The connection with acute, short-lived conditions becomes hard to see. But irritable bowel, colitis ('bowel-itis'), and its intestinal relative Crohn's disease (or regional ileitis), nevertheless originate in this way. They are all milestones on a slippery slope towards worse and worse trouble.

BACK TO THE SOIL

The hazards and insecurity of hunting and fishing were more than compensated by the hugely increased mobility and range they made possible. But the uneasy adaptation of our basically vegetarian system made heavy reliance on meat essentially a temporary phase, and a stepping stone to something better.

So the invention of agriculture – perhaps 100,000 years ago – was a very significant advance, especially the discovery and breeding of crops whose fruit can be successfully stored throughout winter. By far the most successful of these were the cereals, developed by selective breeding of grasses to produce bigger seeds.

Many crops produce storage organs underground – such as potatoes, carrots and turnips. But they are vulnerable to attack by rodents, insects and moulds, which digest the stored starch rather easily. Consequently, they cannot be relied on to survive an entire winter in storage above ground.

This is because of the way energy is stored in these roots. It is made during summer in the plant's leaves in the form of sugars, which are compacted by stringing them together as starch. The starch in plants of this kind is jointed like the branches of a tree, with many loose ends available to be unpicked. Consequently, the digestive juices of all manner of creatures, including moulds and other germs, can release the sugars quickly and easily. Preventing spoilage by moulds would have been largely beyond the capabilities of our Iron Age ancestors.

The special secret of cereal starches is that they form one long daisy-chain without branches, leaving only one end loose to be unpicked. That long string is then spun into a tiny grain, like a ball of knitting wool, with the workable loose end outermost. This means that only one digestive enzyme can work on each microscopic grain of starch, which therefore takes many hours to dismantle into sugars. Only larger creatures such as insects and rodents can do this successfully, so problems of spoilage in store are easier to prevent.

There is, however, a snag to this. We have almost as much difficulty in dismantling the starch as moulds do! To cope with this we invented a wide variety of ways of cooking cereals to open up the starch grains and make them more digestible – bread, cakes and porridge that soften and swell the grains, and biscuits that crack them open. Even so, cereals remain the most indigestible of our foods, partly because of their obstinate structures and partly because they are so new. We have not had much time in which to practise getting round them.

SECRET WEAPON

History has only been recorded for about 10,000 years and all we have discussed so far is prehistory. I have speculated about the stages at which our bowels and stomachs became necessary and may have evolved, safe in the knowledge that no one can really prove or disprove my contentions. My next step is bolder and may seem quite outrageous, but you will be able to test the truth of it for yourself.

We humans have not only one stomach, but effectively two.

The second stomach is our most recent adaptation, probably in the last 50–100,000 years. It enables us to cope with cereal starches. It represents a functional adaptation, not a radical mutation. This failure to fit with fashionable genetic theories is probably why we have not credited it before.

Surgeons call it the fundus, or upper part, of a single stomach. It is perfectly true that the stomach at rest is a single, kidney-shaped organ – as depicted in every drawing in any other book you will ever see. And of course surgeons only work on resting stomachs – remember the 'nil by mouth' at the foot of every bed!

The fundus is an upward and sideways swelling of the *cardia*, or main portion of the stomach. Once meat is smelt or chewed, however, the fundus discharges the juices required for digesting it, but cannot itself tolerate them. Instead they gather in the lower part or pyloric antrum, next to the exit valve of the organ, whose lining is sufficiently well defended by abundant mucus production from being digested by mistake.

The stomach begins to elongate dramatically, often reaching four times its normal resting size. Once the meat is swallowed it collects in the enlarging pyloric antrum, which massages and folds it by muscular contractions to mix in the juices – and incidentally to keep the whole brew a safe distance from its own skin.

Meanwhile the fundus stands by, completely passive. A muscular purse-string constriction tends to form across the top of the antrum, but does not really tighten up unless starchy food is eaten in a later course of the meal. This requires prolonged digestion with the saliva, the mucus liquid that moistens our mouths. The mixing takes place in the mouth, and calls for prolonged chewing – which both breaks down the cereal seeds and calls up plenty of saliva to mix with them.

By the time each mouthful is swallowed it has been softened, but not liquefied. It is held in the fundus, completely separated from the antrum. The fundus becomes a holding vessel, giving the time required for the entire cereal portion to be digested into sugars and liquefied. This is about the same time that meat requires for its entirely different digestive process, going on simultaneously in the pyloric antrum. By the time both processes are finished, the load from each vessel is ready for onward transit to the intestine.

This whole sequence of events can be seen on barium x-rays of even the fasting stomach. Yet radiologists do not comment on it, surgeons ignore it, and nutritionists completely fail to grasp its significance – if they even know it happens. It is the basis of the trick that cured the helicopter pilot whose story I told in the previous chapter. And my knowledge of it stems entirely from the acute observation and curiosity of just one man – Lionel Picton – whom I also introduced in the last chapter.

It has enabled humans to become, from the dietary point of view, the most adaptable and efficient species on earth. This was the basic necessity that underwrote all other developments. These burgeoned as soon as we had settled and begun to grow food from year to year, storing it reliably, preserving ample seed to plant in succeeding springs, planning accurately for future needs. We were no longer totally preoccupied all winter with surviving until spring.

It is no accident that elaborate social structures, written language, mathematics, architecture, religion, arts, science and technology began to develop wherever cereal grains were efficiently exploited. In the tropics it was maize. Everywhere else cereal grains underpinned the civilisations that dominated the temperate regions. Wheat, being the most nutritive, was the most successful. Even in China, large amounts of wheat are cultivated along with the less nourishing rice. Wherever wheat could not thrive, less demanding crops – oats, barley or rye – took its place.

How extraordinary it is that the secret underpinning the existence of all this history should have been so utterly forgotten. The mistakes that followed were inevitable and disastrous. Until we had penetrated to this, the heart of the matter, we could never have appreciated fully the awesome, blundering, simple stupidity of it all.

Unfortunately that is not the end of it. A strong undercurrent to all this development, from its very beginning, is the mystery of how we pick out our food from the enormous range of less nourishing – even poisonous – possibilities available. Which deserves an entire chapter of its own.

Chapter Four: Our Waste of Taste

I started my study of physiology in 1963, at a very prestigious university department packed with great names. By that time a good deal was known about how nerves and muscles worked, about hearts, kidneys, blood and respiration. We knew something about the senses of touch, hearing and vision. Many of these functions had been worked out by former and present members of that department, and the history of these discoveries was related with justified pride.

When it came to the senses of taste and smell, however, the mood was rather different. I vividly remember our young lecturer's vivacious, sharp-witted approach, and his growing reputation as a bright new research star. He told us what we knew then about the working of the nerve endings in the tongue and nose, and their measurable capabilities. But he contrasted these with the extreme sensitivity and subtlety of taste and smell even in humans, let alone animals like the dog, who are even better endowed. He was candidly at a loss to explain the discrepancy between what he and his colleagues could measure, and what people could do.

My daughter recently completed the same course at the same department, nearly forty years later. Impressive advances in knowledge and thinking had taken place on many subjects; but we still cannot fathom the senses of taste and smell.

It is currently fashionable to stress the need to drink plenty of water, and to define to the nearest gram the portions of each kind of food we daily require to survive in health. It is very odd that we should have to talk about such basic things at all. A dog can drink thirstily and at a great rate, then stop in an instant, having drunk exactly the amount of water he requires throughout his body. No hesitation, no slowing down, no careful weighing of the last few drops. Physiologists already knew forty years ago

Thinking in Mouthfuls

Experiment One

Open a bag of your favourite sweets, and start eating.

How great is the impact in your mouth? Tick the grade.

How many do you fancy? Tick the bag size.

Change to a bag of your favourite soft fruit (cherries, strawberries etc.)

How great is the impact in your mouth? Tick the grade.

How many do you fancy? Tick the bag size

Which had the greater impact? – *tick*   sweets ☐   fruit ☐

Which can you eat more of? – *tick*   sweets ☐   fruit ☐

Experiment Two

Imagine baking two fresh potatoes in the oven. You eat one for lunch today, let the other cool and keep it in the fridge overnight. You then reheat it for lunch tomorrow.

Which potato tastes better? – *tick*   Today's ☐   Tomorrow's ☐

Experiment Three

Imagine yourself eating raw peanuts. Notice the taste.

How many can you eat? Tick the bag size you fancy.

Now imagine raisins mixed with the peanuts. How does that alter things?

Tick the bag size you fancy now.

Now change to salted, roasted peanuts, eaten on their own.

Does that alter your appetite?

Tick the bag size you fancy now.

Contrast your appetites in these three cases. Which can you eat most of?

Which least?

Experiment Four

Imagine drinking from a litre carton of ordinary orange juice, the cheapest available from your supermarket, the type made by diluting concentrated juice from more than one country.

Notice the impact in your mouth. Tick the grade that applies.

How much of the litre could you drink in one sitting? Mark the level.

Now imagine instead a litre bottle of freshly squeezed whole orange juice – about twice the price in the shop. (If you've never bought it, squeeze a whole fresh orange from your fruit bowl and actually taste the juice.)

Grade the impact in your mouth

How much of the litre could you drink in one sitting? Mark the level.

Which had the greater impact? – *tick*   Carton ☐   Bottle ☐

Which could you drink more? – *tick*   Carton ☐   Bottle ☐

the precision with which the drink matches the dog's need. How he does it baffled them then, and still does.

Why we humans do not now seem capable of the same exactitude with water, let alone with food, physiologists have no idea. They hardly even discuss it. Can we always have been so clueless? If our noses can detect as little as a single molecule of some substances in the air about us, surely we are capable of similar instinctive precision about the quality and quantity of what we eat and drink! Our ancestors must certainly have got more out of their taste buds than we do now. Otherwise some unlucky choices, at any time in those thousands of centuries of blind tasting, would surely have killed them off.

The nice thing about food and drink is that we can all experiment on ourselves. You do not even have to move a muscle. Just exercise your imagination on a lifetime's experience, in what Edward De Bono calls thought experiments. A few for you to try are on page xx. It would be too much to expect us to agree about everything, but let's compare notes.

Experiment One: My favourite fruit are blackcurrants, which have an awesome mouth impact even in small quantities. I could only manage a small bag in one sitting. Sweets are rather nauseating after a binge, but they're very more-ish.

Experiment Two: Today's potato wins by a mile. It conveys a full, indefinable satisfaction, whereas tomorrow's tastes bland and merely fills a space.

Experiment Three: Raw peanuts are rather boring: I don't want many of those.

With raisins they are much more interesting; I could manage at least three times the quantity – which includes quite a lot more of the peanuts.

But I could go on eating roasted salted peanuts as long as supplies last.

Experiment Four: Fresh juice has a far greater impact in my mouth – almost explosive, and definitely not quaffable, when compared with reconstituted concentrate. If you ever consume fresh oranges or juice in a country that produces them, the impact is greater yet.

Somewhere in all this I hope you noticed that the amount of a particular food that it takes to satisfy you varies a lot, according to the taste and how it is prepared. Plain items, such as peanuts, often taste better in combinations; but even some quite pronounced flavours – like sweets, salted nuts or carton juice – fail to satisfy you well, in any quantity. You are more likely to stop eating because you feel unwell, than out of real satisfaction.

The two potatoes are the purest test. It's even worth making the experiment in real life, and getting other members of your family to compare, blind, yesterday's reheated potato with a fresh one cooked today. I doubt if any of them would fail to spot the fresh one, yet they would struggle to explain exactly why. The fresh one just tastes more wonderful and interesting, the reheated one rather flat and starchy by contrast.

I find it helpful to set up two scales for the satisfaction I get from different tastes. There's a sideways scale, on which I can rate how filling something is. Both potatoes would make the grade. Then there's a downward scale, on which I rate how deeply satisfying it is. Only the fresh potato passes that test.

In my experience, fresh food items invariably satisfy me deeply, as well as filling me quite quickly. Some of them, like oranges and blackcurrants, are so intensely satisfying that I can only bear tiny morsels in my mouth – the flavour explodes in all directions, jerking everything awake.

For our honeymoon my wife and I visited a farm and restaurant in Ireland that has since become world famous. The proprietor made her name by gathering the best produce she could find from the surrounding farms and fisheries, and cooking it simply but wonderfully. We could only find space for two meals a day – breakfast and either a buffet lunch or a five-course dinner. At all meals we could have as much to eat as we liked, and did not hold back. During the days we explored the neighbourhood gently on foot, but cannot claim to have been heroically athletic. I spent hours each day on a water-colour painting, which did not even involve sitting out of doors.

We were quite sure that, after a week of such gross self-indulgence, we should have gained pounds in weight. When we got home we climbed on my surgery scales with some foreboding. Imagine the surprise with which we registered the news – we had each lost nearly half a stone!

Stunned, we tried to work out what we had been doing so right. In the end the truth dawned, and it changed our lives. We had been so deeply satisfied by everything our hostess had put

before us that we had not actually eaten all that much of it. No
wonder she could afford to be so generous with second helpings
– nobody managed more than token amounts.

Almost immediately we made plans to move to our present
rural home, where we could hope to grow and eat that well for
the rest of our lives.

SENSE AND SENSIBILITY

Even after all these years of practice tasting it, I still find it hard
to put my finger exactly on the difference freshness makes to
food. Words fail me. It relates to quality rather than to quantity –
that much is certain. Quality is the ineffable feature Robert Pirsig
struggled to characterise, throughout his writing and academic
life. We cannot put words to it, but we know it when we see or
taste it. It is, in other words, susceptible to experience but not to
measurement.

That is why modern scientists are so nonplussed by our special
senses. Their mechanisms can be defined, but their sensibilities
cannot. These seem to occupy an altogether higher and finer
realm, where different rules appear to apply.

Actually, when you cast your eyes about you, the whole of
nature seems to be that realm. We are stirred by beauty in a
landscape or object without being able to define it: that's quality.
We marvel at the shapes and forms produced by the different
species of living thing – quite beyond the scientist's comprehen-
sion: that's quality, too. Thanks to David Attenborough and
others like him, we gape with wonder at the ways different
species adapt to each other in their special surroundings –
whether by camouflage or exploitation: quality, once again.

It occurs to me that, laid on top of the physics and chemistry
of the materials in nature, we have another scheme at work. The
relationship is like the one between roads and airways – they
operate the same landscape, but using completely separate
rules.

Some authors have been bold enough to define the separate
dimensions by which quality may be 'measured'. Williamson
contrasted the space–time of quantity with memory–will in
quality – a radically different notion invoking consciousness and

mindfulness as essential features of quality. It rings true: qualities always seem to stir, arouse, or make your spine tingle. It's as if something is being awakened or revived, from numbness through pins and needles to complete delight.

Steiner agreed about the mindfulness and went further, describing not one but several extra layers or bodies, superimposed on each other – like roads, then airways, then space orbits and so on. He supposed each one to be lighter and finer than the next one down, with our physical material the heaviest and coarsest. He described the physical, mental and spiritual characteristics bestowed by each one. Fanciful as this may sound to modern minds, its results in practice are spectacular. I cannot help thinking how much better our education, medical and social systems would be, had we paid more attention to his ideas.

I do not suppose I can help you fully to grasp what these and others have suggested. It is a rather broader topic than the scope of this book. But it is obvious to me that the higher realm or realms we struggle to describe contain the rules by which each species organises its form and its relations. The realm of quality contains the blueprints of life.

What about genes, you may ask. Genes define the chemical workings of a single cell. The genes in every cell of the same body are identical – every cell gets the same chemical instructions. How, then, can different cells know how to be different? How does the skin on your nose know to be different from that on your palms, or on the backs of your hands? How do bone cells in your spine know to make vertebrae, whereas in your leg they make a thigh-bone?

You have to imagine they can read a map, cast invisibly around the body: you could say it is part of your 'soul'. This map is a whole, defining your form and characteristics in complete detail. Each cell can read the fragment of the map that lies over it, and follows the instructions it finds there. You could say that the cell shapes itself to match the invisible shape it reads in the map. So all your cells together create a kind of sculpture, representing in visible flesh the invisible map defined in your 'soul'.

Fanciful? – not at all. Electronic engineers, such as Roger Coghill and Cyril Smith, can even tell us how it may be done. They say the coiled shapes of genetic strings – chromosomes –

make them capable of receiving broadcast waves in a certain range of wavelengths. They also tell us that holographic fields – called scalar fields, containing shapes and information rather than forces – might well 'broadcast' on about that wavelength. What is more, these fields have a colossal capacity for information – far more than enough to spell out each cell down to the finest detail.

A few exceptional biologists take up this theme. Rupert Sheldrake has designed experiments which prove that some such shaping influence – he calls them collectively morphogenetic fields – not only moulds individuals, but is shared in a general way by all the members of a particular species. Your human form is, according to him, defined by the human field shared and evolved by all human beings collectively, down the ages. Your unique individual characteristics are expressed by personal mod-ifications of the collective human field, inherited from your ancestors and superimposed on it.

Some very exciting possibilities arise as consequences of this idea. In the first place, it becomes possible to understand how complex talents and characteristics such as musicianship, or a striking facial resemblance, may be handed down from genera-tion to generation. Genes clearly cannot explain such whole-person characteristics at all. Yet they quite clearly are passed on, by some means or another.

Secondly, your 'soul', with its dynamic, holographic map of you, is clearly the most permanent thing about you. It endures for generations, whereas the flesh constructed from its blueprint only lasts a few months or years before being replaced. At last we can begin to understand how your photograph remains uniquely you for decade after decade, yet ages gradually too: your 'soul' is holding everything together, despite the gradual march of time.

Thirdly, what is true of the generations of your family holds equally well for the descent of humankind over geological time. Morphogenic fields can evolve intelligently, responding to hap-penings around you. It really is possible that the giraffe stretched his neck simply by wanting to reach high branches, without any blundering help from gene mutations. After all, practically all the genes are the same in most animals, yet the animals themselves differ strikingly. A second, far quicker and more intelligent evolutionary process alongside genes makes it all much easier to credit: you no longer have to suspend your disbelief in the name of science.

This lends credibility to my speculations in Chapter Three. I shall use it remorselessly also in the Second Movement, looking in more detail at the way our intestines are shaped and how they work. The real possibility that your 'soul' carries a blueprint capable of choosing how to evolve makes my whole line of reasoning entirely plausible.

BLUEPRINT IN DISTRESS

Finally, we have hit upon a further mechanism that could cause disease. Suppose that, despite its robust resistance to wear and tear down the generations, your 'soul' took a serious knock. It would probably be chronic rather than short lived, because we are quite good at resisting the effects of short, sharp shocks. So it might be a chronic infection, or chronic poisoning, or prolonged environmental hardship.

In the same way that an antique piece of furniture gathers scratches and chips as it ages – the dealer's 'distress marks' – your 'soul' can gather glitches too. They would have to be subtle because anything major would so much disrupt your design that you would drop dead on the spot. Nonsurvivable damage to one's 'soul' causes death 'of a broken heart' – we know it happens, you see: we just don't realise what it means.

Let's get back to the smaller glitches. These would mislead the way your body shapes, or how it functions, from that point on. You would work hard to keep up the mistake, because it's written into your design now – how could it be wrong? You could even pass this on to your children, along with your talents and facial features; presumably these glitches become just as resistant to wear and tear as the unblemished design.

It's quite commonplace in the experience of any doctor who tries to help people improve their fitness and diet that, as their bodies get cleaner, the disease gets more conspicuous. This makes doctors wonder sometimes whether their patients want to continue being ill; and perhaps some do value the clear identity disease bestows. But most are simply making it biochemically easier for their glitches to shine through. As their bodies become more chemically efficient, they copy more faithfully both the original design and all its blemishes.

Samuel Hahnemann, the originator of homoeopathy, recognised this stubborn tendency to get ill repeatedly in the same way. He called the glitch responsible a 'miasm'. There are miasms resulting from parasitic infestations like tuberculosis, syphilis, gonorrhoea, malaria – all the ancient epidemic diseases that, in some combination, affected most of our ancestors. They did not pass us down the germs, but they have bestowed the miasms. And, thanks to Hahnemann and his therapeutic legacy, miasms can be cured.

Homoeopathic remedies are a great vexation to most of the medical profession. Randomised controlled trials of their effect, the least disputable sort of evidence you can get, demonstrate clear benefit. Even systematic reviews of large numbers of these trials – the last court of scientific appeal – confirm their positive results. Yet according to pharmacology (the chemistry of drugs) there's nothing in a homoeopathic remedy that could possibly do anything at all. It's just a drop of water, or a pellet of milk sugar.

What the doctors are missing is the whole business of 'soul' activity. Far from being fanciful, this must behave like any other commodity – just subtler and finer, as Steiner asserted. It would appear that, in the process of dilution and vigorous shaking by which homoeopathic remedies are traditionally made, the physical substance on which the remedy is based can be discarded, leaving only the blueprint influence still locked up in the solution. This must be something like the truth, because you can dilute a substance to the point where most samples of the solution do not even contain one molecule of the original – yet the homoeopathic potency gets greater, the more you dilute.

So, if your 'soul' has a miasm that matches the special strength of some other creature or substance in nature, the homoeopathic remedy from that material can be expected to 'repair' the miasm – permanently. Not all homoeopaths would agree with this proposition: most stick to matching remedies only to symptom patterns and personal characteristics, which is not so permanently effective nor so deeply working. But to my mind the fact that miasms can be cured – neatly, safely and economically – is one of the chief benefits that homoeopathy has to offer. ('Useful Addresses' contains more details.)

Meanwhile let's return to the question – how do homoeopathic remedies work? Fairy tales often contain important truths, and more often still offer convenient similes. A homoeopathic remedy behaves in exactly the same way in a pellet of sugar, as the genie locked up in Aladdin's lamp. It stays conveniently in long storage, susceptible only to radiant influences like your transistor radio or shaver socket. Otherwise it retains all its powers until rubbed, when it escapes.

You can do this accidentally, by handling the tablet before putting it in your mouth: all the benefit is gone into outer space, without helping you at all. If you open the remedy container to a strong smell, however pleasant, you corrupt it. Or you can confuse everything by mixing the remedy with the taste or smell of food or drink, taken too soon before or after.

I expect by now the penny has dropped. Homoeopathic remedies enter the body in exactly the same way as the essence of your food – via the sense of taste. We come at last full circle, back to our central topic.

TASTE THE QUALITY

Every living thing possesses a quality-body or 'soul', surrounding and arranging its substance. Your sense of taste is part of that, not a matter of quantity at all. It follows, does it not, that what you taste is the quality of what you eat – not its quantity. My depth-gauge, for grading the satisfaction I get from food, is really a quality-gauge.

In other words, food offers homoeopathic effects as well as nutrients.

So the difference you sense between a fresh and a stale potato is determined by the fact that the latter has lost its quality. Living things retain their quality like a sort of capital reserve, treasured up in their flesh. Cooking the flesh kills it and releases the quality. At first it glows brightly, easier to taste than it was in the raw item – you would not at all have fancied eating the raw potato! Eventually, after just a few hours, all the quality has gone.

The deep flavour of a live or freshly cooked item comes from catching most of this radiant quality, enclosed inside your mouth. Chewing up a piece of food has the same effect as cooking – it disrupts the physical structure of the food and releases the quality locked up in it. Either way, the radiance released gets way beyond your tongue and nose to your brain, your pituitary gland, and your thyroid – all nearby. Where exactly you sense the satisfaction is hard to say, because your own quality absorbs the radiance instantly, as a whole. One thing

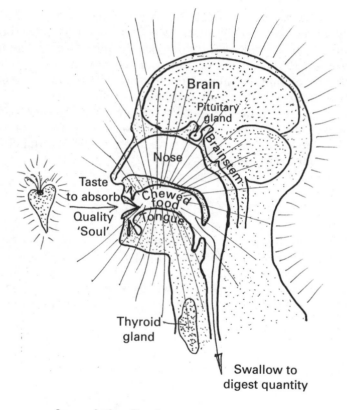

Appreciating Food
The separate paths by which we
take in the 'soul' *quality*
and nutritional *quanitity*
of what we eat

is certain: you have far more at your disposal than just the nerve-endings in your tongue and nose.

Eventually your pleasure at eating each successive mouthful of any fresh item begins to wane. This corresponds with the extent to which your own quality is restored to perfection, by what you have eaten already. Your appetite is as keen as your need for quality, and focuses on the precise food that can give you the quality you need. Once your quality is fully restored, your appetite is zero. This can happen, with practice, between one mouthful and the next.

And what about the quantity? In all living things that have grown naturally, quality breeds truly down into quantity. In other words, tastes faithfully relate to the physical nourishment available. If you have satisfied your needs for quality, then it follows automatically that your physical nourishment is perfect. You can know this immediately – long before each particle of food has been digested, metabolised and located, hours later, in some cell or tissue that needed it.

So it is that taste and smell not only equip us to appreciate food, but to select what we need. We relish far more a food we have long missed than something we ate only hours ago, and as we continue to eat something wonderful the relish gradually fades – even to distaste, in the end.

This is something we still have instinctively as children, part of our innate survival equipment. Our earliest food is, after all, drawn straight from mother's living blood. Later, if we are lucky, we get living milk direct from her breast. It comes naturally to use the same appreciative faculties eventually on an array of fresh finger-foods, all whole-food items prepared simply – if mother has the confidence to arrange things that way, when weaning begins. If we were to analyse the foods selected in this way by a small child it would prove to make up a perfectly balanced diet, just as it does for animals living in the wild.

USE IT OR LOSE IT

A toddler knows nothing about food apart from whether or not he relishes the taste. If the taste is misleading, the equipment does not work. The toddler on ice-cream, sweets, salted nuts or other manufactured, refined or preserved foods, knows no better than you do when to stop – because there are no quality signals to guide him. The diet he selects is unbalanced and probably makes him sick.

Food manufacturers have learned to exploit the relatively crude nerve sensors in our tongues which distinguish salt, sweetness, sourness and bitterness. They are all the equipment we have for coping with food without quality. These flavours can be added to any old junk left over from a more profitable food process, and make it crudely appealing. It is a positive advantage to the manufacturer that the consumer has no means of knowing when to stop eating it.

If you grow up mainly eating foods of this kind, you quickly forget what you are missing. Even if you occasionally experience something with real quality you will have lost the means of appreciating it. Tasting must be practised: use it or you lose it.

Our instinctive taste for quality has built into it the wisdom of ages. It made our remotest ancestors hunger for good things and avoid those capable of harm. Its promise breeds true, right to the smallest detail. Something that honestly tastes good, is good, right down the line. It locks on to the intimate adaptations we have made, to anything natural we have grown up alongside, since the earliest ages of humankind.

Modern departures from this are something else again. They take us right outside the range we can instinctively know to be safe. Rudderless in an unnatural world without familiar quality signals, we become reliant on new-fangled nutritional sciences – the only information and warnings we are going to get. Since most of these experts are employed to work on behalf of the manufacturers of these foods, we can hardly expect them to tell us the unvarnished, awful truth – even if they recognise it.

But our guts can tell that something is up. They rebel, recoiling uncomfortably from a counterfeit that is obvious to them, if not to us. Here is another reason for the lining skin to inflame, with no more hope of respite than we found in the previous chapter. We need to look closely at the many modern intruders that provoke this rebellion. Know your enemy.

Chapter Five: Ration Roulette

It always dismays me to relate the story of what we have done to our food in the past two centuries. I fully realise that there probably never was a completely idyllic era, when our food was plentiful and perfect. No doubt gourmets in every age have bewailed losses they have known since their youth, from the larders, kitchen gardens and tables of their times. But something far more dangerous began to happen during the Industrial Revolution, whose momentum may have slackened marginally in the past decade, but whose consequences will continue to pile up for a long time yet. Globalising tendencies such as the Common Agricultural Policy and the General Agreement on Tariffs and Trade add a twenty-first century spin, which can only make things worse.

You could skip the heart-sink of this chapter and go straight to more positive things in the next, but I advise you to stay with it. In order to dispose entirely of a problem, you need to understand it utterly – otherwise it will simply bounce back in a new form you do not recognise. Know your enemy. And besides, I have to endure the protracted pain of writing it down, and really do not see why you should be spared the brief agony of reading it.

OLD TIMES

Most historians, even those who detail everyday things, do not refer much to the food and eating habits of ordinary people. It is clear, however, that since mediaeval times, the English peasantry subsisted largely on what they could produce or trap around their homes – the 'cottage economy', leading features of which were documented in detail by William Cobbett in 1823. Pigs and chickens figured well in times of prosperity, but not when food was scarce – their owners' desperate needs left little over for livestock. People fell back on cabbages, leeks, parsley and other home-grown vegetables, once the grain harvest had run out. In a bad year that might be during winter, and even wild game would be scarce and overhunted. With luck the grain would last until the summer, when vegetable patches yielded best. But we have noted already how hard it must be to work on a diet only of greens! By Cobbett's time turnips had appeared to provide a little energy, but potatoes would only have reached the tables of the better off.

Clearly the harvest was a time of great relief, marked by feasting. Christmas was the excuse to eat whatever livestock the family could not expect to feed through the winter. By Easter, on the other hand, the winter privations were over and whatever seed had not been sewn could be eaten, in confident expectation of easier living for the next few months.

By the fourteenth century methods were well developed for preserving the spring flush of milk from cows and ewes. Butter and cheese could be put aside for the following winter, when milk yields disappeared. Meat could be cured, or salted away in barrels. Sugar and honey were scarce, so sweet preserves were yet to be invented; but pickling in vinegar would have been possible, using beer that had gone wrong or been deliberately aerated. Most fruit was therefore eaten fresh, between the Lammas harvest (at the beginning of August) and Christmas (at the end of December).

Plainly, peasants were not tempted with anything very rich for very long. They had, nevertheless, to survive the filth of their immediate surroundings, as well as plague and pestilence brought in by visitors, and raids by warlike neighbours. Life was hard, insecure and short.

The advent of international trade introduced to the markets new vegetables such as the potato; wines and exotic nuts and spices. These were, however, expensive and beyond the reach of the poor. Even the growing urban classes could not afford large supplies.

By the eighteenth century tea, chocolate and coffee were popular social drinks and sweetmeats were more plentiful, thanks to large specialist estates in the West Indies and Orient. Tate in Liverpool and Lyle in Greenock received and refined much of the sugar cargo, which was sufficient for the limited needs of a luxury market right into the 1920s.

To do justice to the potential of this product, heavy puddings and cakes were reinforced by new recipes for delicate pastries and confections. For these a finer flour was required, excluding as much as possible of the coarse chaff which comes from the outside skin of wheat seeds. In order to provide this, millers introduced fine screen sieves into their operations as a side-line – fussy to manage, but profitable as a premium-priced specialist item. The chaff, or bran, was sold to livestock breeders and ostlers as a premium feed.

The celebrated Mrs Isabella Beeton gave us some idea of the preoccupation with such delicacies of her well-to-do contemporaries, when in 1859 she set out at length her thoughts on household management. She devoted 827 of the 1,112 pages in my edition to food. Puddings, preserves and confectionery get 24 per cent of that, plus bread, biscuits and cakes another five per cent, second only to meat at 34 per cent. Fish comes in at 9 per cent, sauces pickles and stuffings 10 per cent. Vegetables and soups rate 7 per cent each, and dairy produce only 3 per cent – requiring little preparation for the table.

Meanwhile the masses would, right until the middle of the nineteenth century, have still relied far more on vegetables and bakery. And the cheapest flour they could get – whether from oats, barley or wheat – was always wholemeal.

FOOD GETS INDUSTRY

The really big opportunities to upset this ancient balance of things came first with the invention of steam engines, which encouraged the developments in engineering that by the end of the nineteenth century had revolutionised the milling of flour. The new apparatus was a steel roller device which could mill grain far faster than traditional stone milling, and also separated out its various components automatically without further processing. This made the sought-after white, refined flour far cheaper to produce, which eventually made this prized bakery ingredient more accessible to the public. It also made wholemeal flour harder to reconstitute so that, in a curious reversal of circumstance, this became the more expensive product.

The industries that burgeoned out of this development could see nothing wrong with it, of course. They were able to sell white flour at something approaching the customary premium, though it cost them far less to produce. They could charge extra for the additional work of reconstituting wholemeal, which previously had been the standard product. And they could sell a great deal more bran and wheat germ to livestock fatteners and horse dealers.

Our bodies were not so fortunate. The rough wholemeal grist, on which our forefathers had relied for tens of thousands of years, was much of a piece with the vegetables that had always been our staple before then. They helped to balance up the large meat intake, which by then had become more usual. Indeed, the bran in wheat was particularly suitable for swelling into a bulky, fast-flowing jelly that can ensure a quick passage through the intestines of a heavy meat meal that might otherwise begin to rot inside them.

The sudden introduction of white flour disabled all that: sudden, because it took only 100 years. It requires at least a millennium for us to adjust to anything so dramatic, and the decline in health which resulted may mean we do not have that long.

The fibrous bran was not the only casualty of roller milling. The mineral dust and germ, too, were sacrificed. Wheat germ is the speck of seed substance inside the grain, from which will grow the germinating shoot. The white flour that constitutes most of the grain is only the food store provided to get the germ through its first crucial weeks of development, before roots begin to draw nourishment from the soil outside. The germ is the richest part of the entire seed, with most of its enzymes, proteins and oil – including substances the germ can make but which to us are vitamins.

Germ may be a small part of the whole grain but its disproportionate value is multiplied further by the large contribution cereals make to our food now. We are missing it badly.

The millers have in the past few decades been forced by law to put some of the missing minerals and vitamins back, but not in the same form as they were removed. In nature form is everything, as we began to see in Chapter Four. The purified substitutes provided by twentieth-century chemists for the vitamins and minerals found naturally formed in grains of wheat arouse in our intestines not welcome but hostility.

INDUSTRY GETS CHEMISTRY

Chemistry, too, has ancient roots – the Iron Age – but began to distinguish itself from alchemy during the eighteenth century. It was largely a pastime of those with leisure, one of whom distinguished himself by bringing simple chemistry into the life sciences via agriculture. This man was Justus, Freiherr von Leibig.

Leibig's 1840 account of his most famous experiments would never today have made it past the peer review process, which is intended to weed out bad science before it can be published. He took samples of soil and burned them, ignoring the smoke and paying attention only to the ash. It would be obvious now that what distinguishes soil from powdered rock is entirely in the smoke, but organic chemistry was in its infancy and Leibig commanded a certain respect.

His finding was that, wherever a soil sample comes from, its ash invariably contains nitrogen, phosphorous and potassium – conventionally abbreviated to N, P and K. And these elements would still not have attracted lasting attention, except that adding them to the soil multiplied crops by a factor of ten.

Most things are justified, rightly or wrongly, by their results – especially if profits are included. Chemical fertiliser is still categorised by its NPK content, long after the dramatic initial effect on agriculture has worn off. We now know that extra NPK plundered the organic reserves of the soil, laid down to provide crops in subsequent years. Using NPK is like selling off the family silver. The result is impoverished soil and feeble, defenceless crops that need artificial pharmaceutical protection – insecticides and herbicides – in order to survive at all.

The most serious casualty of this is the mineral content of crop plants, including wheat. The term 'mineral' means 'something mined' – in this context, a food factor that can only be obtained from the soil. Most plants cannot dig for the metals they need without help from fungi that normally wrap round their roots. The fungi, in their turn, need help from germs that live free in the soil. These germs digest crumbs of powdered rock, turning them into a form they can use for themselves and can trade on into the root fungi. The topsoil is really the surface zone where all this is going on. The subsoil is the outermost layer of the geological earth, waiting to be digested into living soil on the earth's surface.

Agricultural chemicals have severely reduced the numbers of both germs and fungi in the soil, drastically limiting the availability of metals to the plants growing above. This is not intentional: crop protection chemicals can also drip on to the soil and kill the organisms there. Dead soil cannot maintain its crumb structure, nor retain half so much moisture, so rainfall starts to

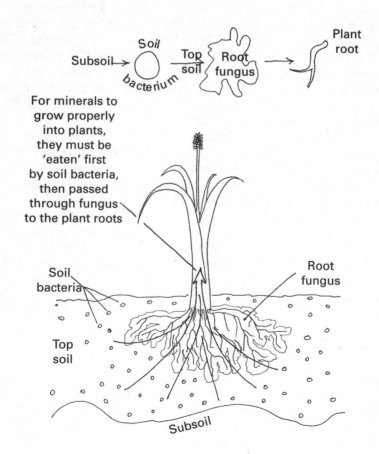

forge runnels across the land, flushing topsoil into the ditches and away.

Farmers and agrochemical companies alike know that all this happens, but so far neither has found a way of stopping it – except abandoning chemical dressings and returning to organic methods. This is not high on the agenda for manufacturers of agricultural chemicals.

Farmers, for their part, face several years growing conversion crops before they can earn the premiums attached to organic food. Having once relied on the expertise of agrochemical representatives, they also find it hard at first to return to making their own unaided judgements. The organic organisations do their best to provide advice but it is no match for the richly funded advisory service available from the chemical companies. Farmers have also usually run up considerable debts to obtain the large agricultural machines necessary to mass-produce crops chemically, all on the assumption that larger profits would pay them off: They have grubbed out hedges to create the prairies on which these machines operate to best advantage, exposing the soil to winds which whip up dust and blow it away, accelerating the soil erosion.

The public reaction against genetic manipulation of farm seed, together with the severe downturn in farming fortunes during the past decade, have made the organic option attractive to many more farmers now. Even quite large land holdings are being quietly converted to organic standards, producing more thatcher's straw (one of the permitted conversion crops) than anyone can use at present. Nevertheless, it will be years before this brings back sufficient minerals into their produce. Soil takes only a few years to destroy, but most of a century to rebuild in full. A complete mineral complement will be one of the last features to return to the future organic crops from once-chemical land.

Meanwhile it is almost impossible to put together a diet with adequate mineral content in the right form for human health, because every available ingredient – apart from seafood – is itself deficient. Intensive agriculture with the plough was enough to lower food minerals by up to 25 per cent, even quite early in the twentieth century. The addition of NPK fertilisers pushed that up to nearer 40 per cent on average. Now, with soil damage from crop protection chemicals, the mineral loss ranges up to 80 per cent in the most intensively farmed areas. Even heavy reliance on food from the sea cannot put such a severe imbalance right.

Besides these deficiencies there are hidden extras in modern food – residues of the sprays themselves. Most of them don't wash off with water. They dissolve only in fat or detergent – quite deliberately, to penetrate the fatty shells of beetles and bugs. Fat-soluble poisons are the hardest for us to get rid of too: our bodies run mostly on watery solutions. When we eat even small amounts of pesticides they first kill off some of the harmless and helpful germs lining our intestine and bowel; then irritate the skin lining the intestines themselves. Having been absorbed into the body they tend to accumulate in fatty tissues over the years – not just blubber but the lining skins of cells, which contain many fatty substances too. As the concentration of agrochemical builds up, it can eventually reach levels which, though still quite low, begin to interfere with the function of those cell membranes. In other words, chemicals that kill very small creatures can also harm us, by accumulating in our bodies gradually over the years.

The bottom line of all this is perhaps the most serious effect of all – the general devitalisation of food crops. Living, well formed food participates fully and well in the economy of the intestine and bowel; encouraging the right germs to form and deterring the wrong ones, cherishing the delicate skin of the intestine and being made welcome. Modern produce would be incapable of that, even if there were no chemical spray residues and no mineral deficiencies – the contrast so clearly illustrated by Pottenger's cats (Chapter Two). The food has not had the opportunity to acquire the structural richness it should achieve, because it cannot sustain the 'soul' to put it there.

Vivid flavour is a prime characteristic of food that has been grown properly – the lesson of Chapter Four. The flabby taste of chemically grown food is its most transparent failure. Yet, unless you have had the opportunity of tasting better, you have no means of judging this. I remember very clearly a salient example. My wife and I had begun our quest for regular supplies of decent food, and found a source of free-range eggs in Lewisham. We sat down to eat one boiled for breakfast the following morning. The first mouthful transported me back thirty years to a first-floor breakfast-room in Bromborough Pool, overlooking the Mersey, where I last ate eggs as good as that. They were laid by hens that scratched for their food among the manure-heaps and pig-sties in the smallholding next door.

I cannot say when that distinctive flavour-in-depth had begun to die. Not suddenly with our move to London: it must have happened gradually as new methods of production were introduced, nationwide. In any case it had completely escaped my notice. But rediscovery of the authentic egg after so long makes you passionately loyal to it ever after. We all urgently need that vivid discovery or reminder, right now. And not just about eggs.

CLOSING IN

Growing up in the Wirral countryside during the immediate postwar years provided other experiences that you cannot so easily acquire now. Eggs were a rather seasonal food, and chicken was rare outside Christmas. Milk changed its character and flavour as the pastures ripened through spring and summer. Orange juice had to be squeezed from the whole fruit, and drunk from tiny glasses – though the flavour was such a punch in the mouth you would not have wanted much anyway. Sweets were still on ration until about 1950, so we simply weren't able to over-indulge.

Little by little since then everything has become available almost continuously, with very little reference to season. The same methods of mass production, that increased yields to match demand, also extended their availability throughout the year. A new postwar ideal was being pursued with enthusiasm, of providing cheap food in abundance.

We have already seen how this weakened its quality and nutritive value, as well as its flavour; but it did more. In the first place, consider some of the methods employed. To get animals to grow faster and put on flesh, antibiotics are added to their feed. This not only alters the bacterial populations of their own intestines but encourages the survivors to develop antibiotic resistance – one of the causes of bowel disease in humans, as we shall see. The hormones used to enhance the milk yield of dairy cattle are equally reprehensible and can have devastating effects in humans, though it is not clear yet that these include intestinal damage. I hardly need add the disaster we still face as a result of the cannibalistic ingredients that were, until recently, permitted in concentrates fed to livestock. We do not, I am sure, yet know the full ramifications of this extremely dangerous practice.

Secondly, the range of food varieties available became far narrower. Where once farmers would indulge their preferences for different types of cattle, different breeds of chicken and vegetables, they gradually standardised on the most prolific types. What is more, these were selectively bred to become yet more intensive, and far more reliant on help from the farmer to survive.

As a result we now find ourselves living on far fewer types of food than we once did, and eating those few types, day in, day out, throughout the year.

The range is alarmingly narrow. I am not sure of their rank in terms of quantity consumed, but here are the main items that come to mind. Wheat and a few other cereals – chiefly maize – head the list, almost always in highly refined forms. Next comes sugar and all its relations – dextrose, glucose, hydrogenated glucose syrup, invert sugar, isomalt and the rest. Then everything from the cow – beef and 'animal fat' as well as dairy produce. Then come chickens and their eggs. The one to watch is soya, now a huge crop from which much vegetable protein is derived. After that come potatoes and other members of that family – tomatoes, sweet and hot peppers, tobacco and aubergines. Then come a large quantity of vegetable fats – largely coconut oil at one time, now more likely 'hydrogenated vegetable oils' processed from rape seed and soya. Citrus fruit juices bring up the rear, but are a significant surge in the diet of Northern Europe.

This may sound a decent range at first, but we have to consider the family groupings as basically one food type. All cereals have been developed from the grass family, and share many features. It is common, in people sensitive to wheat, for other cereals also to provoke a reaction if eaten more regularly instead. The same applies to the many plant foods related to tomatoes – all members of the family *Solenaceae*. In fact, the list in the previous paragraph comes down to only about eight distinct food types.

Why does this matter? Ronnie MacKeith, a late great paediatrician, put his finger on it. We know that people are good at coping with a huge variety of germs in and around our bodies, doing no harm. Reduce the range of varieties by a factor of ten, or make a handful of types predominate, and disease becomes far more likely – even though the total number of germs remains the same. We thrive on diversity, but crumple under intense attack on a narrow front.

Hans Selye cast light on the effect of time on all this. He worked out the nature of stress and its effects on animals. He started with the concepts of stress and strain as developed by engineers. English was his second language and I think he rather confused stress (the challenge) with strain (its effect). Nevertheless, his major contribution was to observe the existence of a threshold, below which a stress does not strain a living thing much at all – it copes by adaptation within its reserve resources. Beyond the threshold reserves run out rather suddenly and symptoms – distress, or strain – dramatically appear.

Selye found that the threshold for tolerating stress depends heavily on the time for which it applies. We can tolerate huge stresses, like a car crash, for a few seconds: but rather weak stresses can upset us if they apply over periods of years.

We can see from all this that a diet including a huge variety of foods, each available during a limited season, is very congenial for human beings. Drastic reduction in the variety, and virtually continuous exposure, create real dangers. The science to prove that came after the event, unfortunately. We shall see the form these dangers take as we follow the journeys through the intestine of different foods, in the next chapter.

E FOR EXPEDIENCE

The rapid increase in food quantity, at the expense of quality and variety, was largely the business of the 1950s. It led inevitably to mass distribution, to the supermarket culture, and a major drive to increase the shelf-life of food products. Equally inevitable, though for social rather than agricultural reasons, was a new demand for quick and easy meal preparation. These two impulses formed an intricately interwoven undercurrent to the next 30 years.

Heat treatment and vacuum-sealing in tin cans was a direct descendant of the bottling technology of Mrs Beeton's day. It was already well established before the Second World War. The new development that swept the 1960s was deep freezing, which became viable with the development of flash-freezing technology on an industrial scale.

Canning has its drawbacks. It contaminates the contents with traces of cadmium near the maximum permitted levels recommended by the World Health Organisation. Heat treatment also devitalises and degrades food, which is obvious when canned goods are compared with the fresh item. But there it ends: unlimited access to prepared foods well out of season seems hugely to outweigh those limitations.

Deep freezing appears to improve on that. It conserves far better the appearance and taste of fresh food, but that is deceptive: the nutritive value of the food after freezing and thawing is reduced by as much as half. This reduces the flavour-in-depth and increases consumption, to which manufacturers and supermarkets have no objection. But deep freezing is the first technology in which flavour is dissociated from true content.

It went on from there. Freeze-drying came next – the production of small packets of desiccated ingredients that would reconstitute quickly with water to produce a semblance of the target food. This could just as easily be minestrone soup as plain garden peas – a great leap forward in convenience, to suit the increasingly busy lives of family caterers. But the cost in this case was far greater. In reality, freeze-drying was not a good enough technology to guarantee acceptable results just with water. You needed emulsifiers, stabilisers and anti-caking agents to make sure the texture reconstituted properly. Colour and flavour did not survive the process too well, so enhancers of both were added to the recipes.

Thereafter creativity knew no bounds. Why stop at chemically simulated versions of traditional recipes? This technology could create something entirely new. Any edible waste from any food process could be treated physically and chemically, flavoured artificially and cooked up into something saleable. This began the explosion of new snacks, confectionery and processed meats that filled the shelves from the 1980s onwards.

None of the chemicals used for these purposes added anything at all to the nutritive value of the product, which remained near zero. They were cosmetics, without which these creations would have tasted as disgusting as they were. Some of the additives were very odd items to find permitted in food at all – dyes, chalk, titanium oxide, aluminium, sulphur dioxide, soap, Epsom salts, chlorine, talc and sand. And although none of them individually amounted to much, together the chemicals eaten daily by the average citizen had reached half an ounce – 13 gm. That is the weight of 23 soluble aspirin tablets.

And that was the touchstone that set off the first signs of a massive public backlash. Food manufacturers had co-operated across Europe in a codification process for food additives that enabled them to be identified in brief on food packaging. The results of this process was the ill-fated list of E-numbers. When shoppers started seeing these numbers on food labels they were not best pleased. The Ministry of Agriculture, Fisheries and Food tried to reassure us by publishing, *Look at the Label* in 1982, a pamphlet that had precisely the opposite effect. I promptly wrote a reply for the Soil Association – *Look Again at the Label* – which criticised strongly the worst offenders. Several books and magazines took up the theme over the next few years, to the extent that products got piled back on the shelves if shoppers thought they had 'too many E's'. Several of the manufacturers reverted to using their long-winded chemical names, as camouflage!

It cannot be said that this reversed the use of artificial chemicals in food products to any great extent; but it checked the trend, and put the innovators on the back foot. Quite possibly the move back towards wholemeal bread gained impetus from the reaction. White flour tolerates a long list of additives that are not permitted in wholemeal, and the general impression of bakers' shop windows has definitely grown browner in the past 20 years. And, just possibly, more people have bought more fresh food items since then, to go with a slightly diminished range of packaged purchases. I certainly hope so, though some of the groaning trolley-loads I follow through the checkouts still make me wonder.

In any case we are still far from undoing the harm done by this move towards fake food. Nor are the innovators deterred. Indeed, their latest baby is their proudest offspring yet.

GM

Genetic manipulation of species is not so new as you may think. Plant and livestock breeders have done it for centuries, by selecting parents with desirable characteristics in the hope of enhancing these in their offspring. The earliest attempts and most successful results, in my opinion, have been the cereal crops discussed in Chapter Two. More modern examples may have diluted nutritive benefit in return for larger crop yield, but in general I cannot say this trend has of itself produced obvious threats to intestinal health.

Much more recently, and rather quietly, bacteria have been genetically altered to produce something desirable as an industrial end-product. This older form of 'biotechnology' has often replaced much more costly, inefficient and polluting processes requiring large, unsightly chemical plants. Arguably it is one of the most wholesome innovations to come out of genetic modification. But you are not invited to eat the altered organisms. What has provoked far the biggest public reaction ever is the gratuitous genetic alteration of plants and animals intended as food. By this I mean the implantation of genes from entirely different species that nature would never have been in a position to accomplish.

The first objection to this practice is the advantage being sought by the manufacturer. The most celebrated example is the modification of soya beans to tolerate far larger applications of a particular herbicide. The herbicide in question is of course another product of the same company. This openly commercial development raises all sorts of ethical issues, which do not bear directly on our present purpose. Much more to the point is that, since these crops will survive more intensive herbicidal dressing, much larger residues will be found in products made from them. These are undeclared, and exacerbate the intestinal problems people already had from smaller exposures to the same herbicide. Where one product has led, others will surely follow.

The second main objection that concerns gut health takes us back to the previous chapter and the subject of formative forces. Genetic manipulation is founded in the belief that genes organise everything about the creatures they belong to. They cannot do so, however, as we have seen. Many changes simply disable the organism from working out its 'soul' at all, which explains the huge number of failed attempts. This is actually quite reassuring to those of us who distrust the entire project – it is probably doomed to failure in the long run.

However, I remain uneasy that these sorcerer's apprentices, who tinker with matters they scarcely understand, may spark off something they do not bargain for. It may radically corrupt appetite and the normal instinctive warnings that accompany taste sensibility, thereby overriding the instinctive protections we currently have against eating the wrong things or too much of the right ones. We very much rely on those instincts to help us eat properly and safely. Natural things that taste good in depth and go down well, guarantee not to harm us. Even chemically manipulated, counterfeit food can be exposed, by comparing its taste with that of the real thing. Genetic manipulation may, conceivably, defy that protection and start to harm us insidiously. The harder and more enthusiastically they try to exploit the technology, the more likely is such a thing to happen.

MEDICINES

All this threatens people who never take a medicine in their lives. But they are now a minority of us. Most people take from time to time something a doctor has prescribed, or that they have bought over-the-counter, with or without the recommendation of a pharmacist. A great many of these have unwanted effects in the gut, some of which take time to recover even after only a single dose.

The worst are antibiotics and antiseptics, which devastate the germs that ought to be thriving in your caecum. This usually causes diarrhoea and irritable bowel directly, and it will persist unless you do something decisive to restore the germs to their proper balance and vigour.

Probably the commonest medicines in general use are pain-killers. Most of these happen also to make the bowel sluggish. Anything related to codeine of pholcodeine – common in cough medicines – constipates many people noticeably after just one dose.

There are many other medicines with similar effects. In fact, if you read the product leaflet carefully it is hard to find any medicines that do not mention the possibility of gut side-effects. Ironically, some of the medicines given routinely to relieve IBS gut spasms can themselves increase the tendency to constipation – robbing Peter to pay Paul.

CASUALTIES

Humans seem fated to learn by our mistakes. Lionel Picton, the Cheshire doctor you have already met, was by 1930 able to make telling observations of the effects upon his patients of modern tendencies in their diets. One by one, vitamins and then minerals were identified as essential nutrients by the diseases caused for want of them, each one thrown into prominence as food refinement took effect. A whole clutch of new diseases were identified as direct results of eating sugar and several more, including appendicitis, emerged as consequences of eating refined food with insufficient fibre.

Just as medicine seemed to have conquered infections, we began individually to lose the ability to control them for ourselves. Hitherto harmless germs, frequently present in the throats and bowels of healthy people, began in the last 20 years to escape from confinement and produce deadly results – septi-caemia, gastro-enteritis and meningitis. Many people think that infections of this kind are somehow implicated in the rise of chronic inflammatory bowel disease, and this could easily be so.

Others are more inclined to blame environmental pollutants for these developments. A new discipline of Environmental Medicine has emerged in the past 20 years, quite rightly pointing out how incompatible with health are the industrial practices now connected with agriculture, manufacture and food process-ing. Attention has ranged across hormones, pesticides and heavy metal exposures as real long-term threats to health, and impressive laboratory facilities and clinical research findings have gained the respect and attention of increasing numbers of doctors.

The first large group of environmental victims are those who have become intolerant of things they consume. I steer you away from the word 'allergy', which I believe still to be quite unusual. Allergy is an abnormal reaction on the part of the consumer to a traditional food, and is usually demonstrable in immunological blood tests. The commonest culprits are strawberries, shellfish, wheat and dairy produce. Some people react badly to any food naturally containing salicylates – the same chemical family as aspirin.

Intolerance is a far wider problem. These are people who are regularly pushed past their stress threshold by one or more things they are exposed to. Digestive symptoms are in any case common in people under excessive stress of any kind, so stresses operating directly on the intestines via food and drink are quick to provoke them.

Some of the provocation comes from remorseless consumption of too few foods, all the year round. Foods to which people are weaned too young are particularly problematic because the infant immune system is not ready for anything foreign until about six months of age. Breast-fed babies have no problem if they are allowed to tackle other foods only when they are ready, but bottle-fed babies often remain clumsy for the rest of their lives about the foods on which they were reared. These include milk and cereal, which frequently give rise to intolerance problems for this reason.

A further group of people react against chemicals commonly found in foods, rather than the foods themselves. This is not at all unnatural; the substances concerned are frankly provocative or poisonous to all of us. People differ, however, in how much they consume and how well they can put up with it. Once pushed past their limit by one substance their tolerance of others is reduced, so multiple intolerances are exceedingly common. These may add to the problems of dairy produce and cereals, both of which are likely to contain herbicide and pesticide residues. Ironically, wholemeal cereals will be worse contaminated in this way, unless they are genuinely organic. A lot of people feel that, because of bad past experiences, they dare not eat wholemeal cereals – which may otherwise, in principle, aid their intestinal recovery enormously. It often transpires that the spray residues are to blame for the adverse reactions: organic wholemeal would be fine.

Next come a list of well known poisons which you may think had long since been eliminated – lead, mercury, fluoride, aluminium and cadmium. You may be surprised at how much lead is still present in older mains water systems, particularly in city centres supplied by soft water, as for example in Scotland. Mercury has been the staple material for tooth fillings for decades. Cadmium is inhaled with tobacco smoke, and eaten with tinned food. It gets into urban pollution if rechargeable batteries are burnt in land-fill sites or incinerators. All these poison accumulatively, and can at some stage in life begin to cause insidious intestinal symptoms.

ALUMINIUM

We have known for many years that food contaminated with aluminium is capable of damaging the gut. It is naturally present in soya beans, which thrive on it: organic soya plants contain even more. The subject was actively discussed during the early twentieth century, after the introduction of aluminium pots and pans. It was contentious, of course, particularly during the mid century when production of aluminium utensils was at its height, because of the commercial implications. Now that their use has waned it is easier to be dispassionate about the issue.

After fairly prolonged exposure to aluminium, most particularly in food, the damage begins to show as mouth ulcers, gut pain or diarrhoea, often misdiagnosed as chronic appendicitis or colitis. When this vanishes after abstinence from aluminium, sometimes after years of suffering, the causal link is clear enough. But sometimes the effect outlasts the physical exposure to the metal, because aluminium is capable of creating a miasm affecting the 'soul' (Chapter Four). This means that your body continues to behave as if affected by aluminium, even after the exposure is removed.

It is very hard to avoid aluminium completely, but knowing where to find it is a good start. Choose take-away restaurants that pack in microwavable plastic, not aluminium. Do not buy cakes, pies, puddings, *etc.*, cooked in aluminium moulds. Avoid any food wrapped in aluminium foil or supplied in containers with foil tops (such as yoghurt). Fruit juices often come in aluminium-lined cartons, beer and soft drinks in aluminium cans. Pub beer may be drawn from aluminium casks. Many teabags have aluminium added in the process of manufacture, so it is safer to use loose tea. Instant coffee often contains aluminium. If booster immunisations are required request them *without* the adjuvant aluminium acetate. Medicines in blister packs may be in contact with aluminium.

Aluminium is used in food processing as a bleaching, emulsifying and raising agent, so avoid products containing E173, E541, E554, E556 which are aluminium and its salts. Most 'table' salts have aluminium added, so use sea-salt. Processed cheeses and soya products contain undeclared aluminium. Do not use antacid tablets or liquids containing aluminium oxide. Aspirin may enhance the absorption of aluminium. Buy toothpaste in a plastic tube. Fortunately most water authorities have switched from aluminium to iron additives, to clear colour from tap-water. A jug filter or reverse osmosis unit removes either.

FLUORIDE

You may be surprised to see fluoride on the list at all. It is supposed to be good for your teeth – helping to prevent the kind of decay that gets you involved with mercury fillings. Fluoride is a long and controversial story. I believe that the chief reason for its promotion is the need to get rid of it as safely as possible. Lots of industries produce it, and would dearly like to be able to sell it on profitably. We are asked to have it in our water, which is a very clumsy way of getting us to consume it but would dispose neatly of all the fluoride in the world. It would also cause major environmental problems, since quite small concentrations of fluoride in rivers, lakes and seas damage the life they support. In any case, whether it is in your water or not, many of us are consuming from other sources more than enough for any benefit there may be, and far too much to be safe from long-term accumulative effects. Apart from the strong concentrations in most toothpastes, fluoride is naturally present in teas from Asia. Just as soya thrives on aluminium though its human consumers don't, tea plants thrive on fluoride.

The most bizarre thing is that in this country doctors cannot test to see whether you are getting too much fluoride. They do not even know what the symptoms of excess fluoride might be. But in India, where tests are readily available and doctors are alert to the problem, intestinal disease is very clearly associated with fluoride consumption. It causes a pain in the stomach which makes the doctor think first of ulcers. When he investigates, however, the problem is not a hole through the stomach lining but general wear, thinning and cracking of the skin cells all over the stomach lining. Very likely the same effects occur further down the intestine, though that is not so clearly demonstrated.

Fluoride may also be one reason for a gradual decline in the working of the thyroid gland, which is getting much more common in younger people. A drop in metabolic rate caused by reduced thyroid action, of any cause, constipates the bowel drastically.

TOO CLEAN

I shall not press on remorselessly with a potentially endless list of bad news items, but there is one more that deserves the prominence of being last. It is ordinary household washing-up liquid, the purpose of which is to dissolve stubborn fatty residues from dirty dishes. It is, unfortunately, just as good at dissolving the delicate fatty lining membrane that we have noted already, on the cells that form the skin of your intestine. If they survive any fluoride you swallow, they will definitely succumb to washing-up liquid – even tiny traces of it.

And it is surprisingly easy to consume. If you do not rinse your pots carefully with clean water before drying them, residues of the detergent cling to the plates and cutlery. From there they get into the next meal served from them, or get swallowed directly from your fork or spoon. Dr John McLaren-Howard, director of a major London medical laboratory specialising in environmental medicine, is astonished at how little detergent it takes to wreck totally a significant number of lining cells in the intestine. With consequences of the kind we shall explore more thoroughly in the next chapter.

Second Movement
Rationale for Recovery

Chapter Six: Read Mark, Learn and Inwardly Digest

It has probably not occurred to you that when you swallow something it does not enter your body. Instead it passes through your gut, the tube from your mouth to your backside. The gut is really a part of the outside. You may choose to absorb into your body some of what passes through your gut, or you may not.

The skin of your gut meets your outside skin in your mouth and around your anal margin, and shares with it one property at least – separating the outside world from your true insides. Otherwise, however, it contrasts strongly. It even arises from an entirely different layer of the embryo that formed you, distinguished from your outside skin at a very early stage. These layers of your embryo were given Greek names, to indicate their fundamentally important difference: the endoderm (inside skin) and ectoderm (outside skin). Broadly speaking, the ectoderm went on to form your skin, eyes and nervous system – everything to do with your awareness of the outside world.

Your endoderm is a little harder to appreciate, but it's worth the effort. Apart from making the skin of your gut, it made most of your internal glands and organs, apart from those to do with your circulation. Your liver, half your pituitary gland, your thyroid and thymus glands, your lungs – all these come from the endoderm.

Whereas your ectoderm deals with the outside world, these hidden endodermal structures are to do with maintaining yourself as a unique, separate 'I'. While ectoderm is extroverted, endoderm is introverted. While ectoderm deals with your material prosperity, endoderm is the agent of your 'soul'. It is deeply involved with your immunity, notably its positive side – your self-assertion. In particular it administers the system whereby all your separate parts, regardless of their separate origins, respond and behave as integral parts of your own whole body.

Let's consider what this means. Food is part of the outside world that you choose to feed on. It has its own immunity, because it too is a living thing with a unique identity. Eating therefore represents a gamble. You are betting your immune system against your food's. In letting it into close contact with the skin of your gut you risk an attack – and sometimes that attack actually succeeds, becomes infection or provokes inflammation. If that doesn't happen you dismantle the food into smaller components by digesting it, and absorb these. But you still have to stop these fragments behaving as part of the creature they come from, and turn them into part of yourself.

This is a process we call assimilation. It is biological rather than chemical, and not therefore considered at all in most modern textbooks of nutrition. It works through your 'soul' – about which, you must realise by now, we have very much to learn.

That's enough abstraction for the present. Let's follow the sequence of a meal in practice, and see how it can go right or wrong.

THE MOOD FOR FOOD

Even before you bite the first morsel, a meal is already well underway. You have thought about what you might fancy, gone out and bought it, stored and anticipated it. You have assembled and prepared the ingredients, enjoying the smell as the dish evolves under your nose. You have probably composed and seasoned the recipe to your taste, whatever the original author may have said.

Appetites are sharpening throughout the household. Someone sets the table, you sit down and the dishes are greeted with approval. The chef glows. Rich aromas escape as portions are given out. Only then do you tuck in.

That build-up to a meal determines how it will go down, and how well it will satisfy you. It has been an integral part of the process of eating almost for ever – at least since our ancestors began hunting or fishing for food, and then cooking it. In the first place, there was the immense relief at the prospect of anything to eat at all. The group may have been hungry for days, managing on poorly preserved scraps and tough roots since the last fresh kill. Not for them the easy drag down to the supermarket, with standard supplies guaranteed week after week.

Taste and smell now seldom play so great a part as they should in this build-up. You cannot select packaged, frozen items on that basis: you have to rely on their remembered reputation. Choice cannot be a vivid new experience each time, just something done by rote.

Once defrosted and in the pot, the aromas are unlikely to be so enticing as they could be: mass-production and prolonged storage both rob their intensity. If you doubt this, take a break in France and try a freshly roasted chicken off almost any market. The smell of the stand is a magnet for miles around. The French still rear much of their poultry on a farmyard basis, letting them feed and exercise in a more or less natural way. The difference this makes to the eating quality is quite stunning, and greatly outweighs the additional cost. No spices or stuffing are called for – the flavour is quite rich enough on its own. You begin to realise why we increasingly feel the need to adorn our dishes with elaborate sauces and seasonings – in search of something, anything at all, to challenge our taste buds.

All this presumes you still have mealtimes, in the traditional sense – and that you prepare the food for them yourself. It has become very easy to go through life for months at a time without really cooking at all. If your habit is to take a meal-pack from the freezer and microwave it for a few minutes, then eat it on your knee in front of the TV, none of what I have conjured up applies.

This does matter, a great deal. Most of life is spent in an active mood, moving about and thinking on your feet. You may have no idea at the beginning of each day whether you will succeed in any or all of the tasks you have set yourself That is not so far removed from the daytime challenges facing our remote ancestors – not sure whether they will track game successfully and manage to kill it without being gored, near enough to home to carry it back.

This mood is very antagonistic to eating. It pours effort into muscles and nerves, leaving your intestines blanched, dry and inert. They cannot be jerked successfully back into activity in a matter of minutes. A totally opposite, passive mood of relaxation, warmth and self-indulgence is called for, as part of which your intestines stir into life at the expense of your muscles and intellect. A mellow, reflective, happy ambience is essential for full digestion and appreciation of any meal.

Until the advent of convenience food, none of this need have been said. Hunter-gatherers could get into the right mood on the way home, carrying the catch. Eating inevitably called for a period of preparation and an agreed mealtime, so the right mood necessarily had time to develop. Fast meals got rid of all that – only 30 years ago – and sabotaged the best chance you have of getting them to go down comfortably.

Restaurateurs understand this very well. However good or bad the fare they intend to put before you, they take care to prepare the atmosphere in their establishments to be welcoming and relaxed, with subtle lighting and pleasing décor. The drinks beforehand are not just a means of making extra profit: they slow you down, give you a chance to catch your breath and relax whilst musing through the menu with pleasurable anticipation. For most people, this is a large part of the added value in eating out.

Once the food appears, you can start to devour it with your eyes. The effort of making a dish attractive to all the senses is not wasted. At your best you are not five senses but one sentient being. The total effect of the dish before you harmonises and focuses all your faculties, on the prospect of making that meal become part and parcel of you.

The care and love with which a meal is prepared for family or friends works wonders, too. Once you realise that there is a 'soul' component in every food, it is not so hard to see how a recipe can aspire to a 'soul' as well. It is then a small step to allow the soul of the chef in, as an utterly magical ingredient garnishing every recipe. No one makes rice pudding the way your mother does.

A MOUTHFUL TO STOMACH

So it is that, long before that first morsel passes your lips, its reception is pre-ordained. You either take the time to savour it, chewing into it tentatively, just fast enough to keep that ineffable flavour coming. Or you are more concerned with getting it down quickly, in a lunch break shortened by overrunning sessions or extra midday commitments.

Slow, appreciative chewing ensures that all the 'soul' quality of the meal gets into you properly, through your sense of taste. That's not only the most satisfying way to eat, but also the least dangerous and most comprehensively nourishing. Meanwhile your salivary juices have plenty of time to mix with each mouthful, softening and pre-digesting as far as they can. Vegetation and starchy items have a chance to begin swelling with moisture to a soft gelatinous consistency, with less risk of damage to the skin of your mouth or tongue from sharp edges. Juices released from fleshy fruits and vegetables are swallowed ahead of the solid parts, preparing your stomach and intestine to receive the solids which then follow. Plainly prepared vegetation of any kind slips through the stomach unhindered, in about the time it takes to say it, and comes to rest in the intestine just beyond.

Once you are well practised at the art of eating, the first forkful of flesh food sets off a new process. Even the thought or smell of it can trigger the transition, sometimes prematurely. Flesh requires digestion in the juices available in the stomach, and these begin to flow while you are chewing the first piece. Pieces of meat, pulped and moistened by chewing, mix with acid juices from the upper stomach and gather in the pyloric antrum (page 78). Little by little a kneading and churning process begins, confirmed as this portion of the meal comes to an end, folding the meat and juices in upon themselves – always inward, away from the stomach lining. That is protected by secretions of mucus from deep in its folds, but cannot stand a direct frontal attack from the acid juice. It is, after all, made of very similar protein to that in the meal, and vulnerable to precisely the same digestive process. Getting it wrong opens up a multitude of unwelcome possibilities.

A common mistake is to eat something excessively sweet, directly into an empty stomach. This sets off the first of Cleave's 'saccharine diseases' (Chapter Two) – a flush of acid juices from the upper stomach, just as if the meal were protein. This is

simply a mistake, triggered by the artificially refined confectionery in a way the unrefined, natural ingredients would
usually not have done. But you are deprived of the means of
recognising refined foods, as we have seen – and this is one of
the consequences.

The sweets cannot use up the acid in any way, except by
stopping dead the salivary juices that would otherwise have
started work on any starchy ingredients. Saliva is neutral in
reaction, neither acidic nor alkaline, and only does any digestive
work so long as this neutrality is preserved.

The situation that develops is an accident waiting to happen.
The acid juices from the stomach have nothing legitimate to do,
but are trapped in the stomach at least temporarily. The sweets
are in there too, no digestion taking place. The entire content is a
far more watery liquid than would normally be the case, and no
amount of mucus can guarantee to keep it from trickling into the
folds of skin. Your stomach does its best, mucus production
going into overdrive. More often than not, it fails.

The results are threefold. Some acid attack reaches the skin of
the stomach, causing it to flair and burn to some degree. That is
called nonspecific gastritis. Some sugars and starch grains get
into the crypts of the skin, where they too provoke a reaction –
this time, more mucus production. Finally, the mucus overactivity spreads from the stomach to other organs capable of
mucus production. All the lining skin of the entire intestine and
bowel is in that category, along with the linings of your lungs,
liver, nose, ears and sinuses. The messages ripple out to them
like jungle drumbeats, through the rather slow tracery of fine
nerve connections that network in the continuous lining skin
connecting them all.

The skin reacts by thickening, each type becoming more
active and producing mucus after its own fashion. The most
familiar result is the congested and running nose, often with
sneezing; but chronic asthma is another form it may take. Mucus
made in the bowel may be passed separately, or mixed with
faeces. The tubular parts of the liver react with a bilious material
that often regurgitates into the stomach, and gives an unpleasant
bitter taste if regurgitated from there into the mouth.

Not all this is likely to happen at once, and because of the
slow transmission of nervous messages in the intestinal skin it

can take time after the meal to develop. The trouble is that meals like this are often repeated many times in a day. It is not just confectionery: sandwiches produce a similar result. In this case any protein content of the sandwich – cheese, peanut butter, sliced meat, yeast extract or meat paste – legitimately calls up acid digestion, but the bread in each mouthful gets nowhere in these circumstances. Again, the acid stops digestion of starch and simply breaks up the crumbs into a wet mess. This weakens the acidity, calling for more acid production and wetting the mass still more. Starch grains and acid may get into contact with the stomach lining and again, nonspecific gastritis can develop. The delicate balance of protein digestion is far too easily upset to risk complicating it in any way, certainly not several times a day.

You will probably get away with a rare mistake, but a regular bad habit creates an abnormal climate. In the stomach, this favours a germ called *Helicobacter pylori* – which is just Latin meaning a coil-shaped germ found in the pyloric part of the stomach. This has been blamed for causing ulcers there, and a rather unpleasant antibiotic and antacid treatment is now customary in an attempt to kill them off and heal the ulcers. Of course the ulcers return, along with the germs, because the germs are not the cause of the problem. It is the disturbed climate – acid digesting the stomach skin – that creates both the ulcers and the germs. You have to sort out your own eating and digestive habits first, which in a few weeks heals both problems. If that treatment could be bottled and sold, drug firm representatives would no doubt be urging doctors to prescribe it.

It is relatively easy to switch off gastritis by blocking with drugs the flow of stomach acid. However, the threat remains as long as the bad eating habit persists, so the prescription is potentially life-long. Meanwhile you are unable to digest your protein food much at all, because for that you need the blocked acid juices. Consequently, that protein goes on down the intestine and bowel, keen to make mischief at every turn. Clearly, there is plenty of room in a long lifetime for a situation like this to go badly wrong. It's far safer, cheaper, quicker and easier to solve the original problem properly.

PUDDING AFTER SAVOURY

To digest protein your stomach enlarges considerably, in proportion to the size of the meal. So long as you give it the chance, that meat will in the course of a few hours disintegrate safely into an inoffensive mass of jelly consistency, the acid gradually neutralising and the enzymes spent.

If now you are still hungry, you can safely eat starchy food to make up your energy needs. You do not have to wait those few hours to find out – your taste senses can make that judgement for you. Once the protein course is safely in place and digesting away, you can start chewing bread, roly-poly pudding or Christmas cake.

There are ground rules, as you may expect. It is best not to drink along with starchy food but to let your saliva do all the wetting. That is because it is the enzymes in saliva that will achieve the digestion of that starch. You cannot afford the mouthfuls to get too wet because you want them to retain a

Contrasting views of stomach function

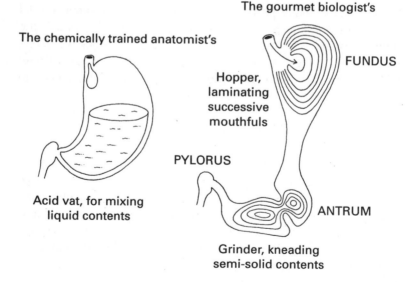

The gourmet biologist's

The chemically trained anatomist's

Hopper,
laminating
successive
mouthfuls

FUNDUS

PYLORUS

Acid vat, for mixing
liquid contents

ANTRUM

Grinder, kneading
semi-solid contents

certain gloopiness – like wet dough, or wallpaper paste. Even without water that is hard if the cereal contains no fibre, which gives rise to the second rule. Eat wholemeal cereals, not refined ones – these become too watery in the mouth and will not do what you need.

If you abide by those two rules, the clever adaptation described in Chapter Three swings into action as you start to swallow the bread. Your stomach elongates further, drawing a purse-string around the top of the pyloric antrum, sealing its contents from a newly fashioned hopper, the fundus of the stomach. No juices are running from its walls now; it receives the gloopy mouthfuls passively, one at a time. Each successive swallow lands a fresh globule on the outside of the last, spreading it out and around the newcomer. In this way a laminated lump builds up, layered rather like flaky pastry. This makes the lump more solid than you would expect from the texture of each globule. So it stays in the hopper, slowly digesting with the saliva, releasing sugars from the chains of starch in each granule.

Depending on your appetite, your stomach just after the meal can be very large indeed – stretching the entire length of your belly, the size of a generous handbag. You should be thoroughly mellow by now, unwilling to move about much – exactly what it takes to preserve the precarious digestive process you have set up. That process also takes several hours, after which time the liquid sugar solution begins to drip through the purse string on to the digested meat below. By then, both parts of the meal are ready for the next stage of their journey, into the intestine.

GUT REACTION

Once you pass the exit valve of the stomach – the pylorus – it is obvious things have changed. All through your mouth, gullet and stomach the skin is relatively thin and flat, as it needs to be to defend itself from a physical injury or digestive attack – the most immediate dangers incurred when you eat another living thing. Consequently, little or nothing is absorbed from there – all the formative forces that make their skin oppose encroachment of any kind.

Beyond the pylorus, the opposite is true. The transition is not immediate, though. The first few inches of the intestine receive through a tube from the liver and pancreas additional digestive juices, which are alkaline and no threat to the lining skin. Thereafter this has long, delicate curtains hanging from it, like seaweed, wafting to and fro in the tide of semi-liquid contents. These are very vulnerable to damage if anything is wrong, but perfectly adapted for the work that now begins – absorption and assimilation of the meal.

An important issue arises here. You spend your entire life keeping other creatures at arm's length, preventing them from colonising your body. However, you also need nourishment, and because we have given up many nutritive jobs that other organisms can do for us (Chapter Three) we have now to eat those organisms. That's pretty sophisticated – holding at arm's length and at the same time letting in.

At birth you cannot yet do this. Feeding only from mother means that you can safely fight off any other creature you may meet, large or small. Only once you have learned to do that confidently, do you dare to explore the sort of food mother seems to like – in the process we call weaning. At its best this is gradual, over many months, during which you get the hang of sorting out admissible friend from intractable foe.

The place where this distinction is made is your sense of taste, picking up on the 'soul' quality of what you are sampling. Some tastes unpleasant or uninteresting, so you don't need that – spit it out. Anything nice you ruminate on in wonder before swallowing.

However, the distinction you made in your mouth only comes home to roost in your intestine, where you have to do it all again. The delicate skin is, incredibly, the front line of your immune system. Not so much the defensive, antagonistic, fortress aspect we think of most easily, but the self-assertive component, responsible for sustaining you. Selecting what you need from the contents of your intestine is relatively easy. Transforming it into part of yourself is a more mysterious art, but much more important. You are capable of absorbing quite large chunks of nourishment, easily large enough to retain some of the identity of the creature you have eaten – especially if it was still alive when you ate it.

The trick is accomplished, of course, by means of a change of 'soul' quality, probably without any alteration to the actual chemistry. This transformation takes place in the cells lining the intestine, that dangle in the delicate veil across your digested meal to make intimate contact possible. The cell 'eats' each morsel – rather like you did, but on a minute scale – and makes the change of identity in its cytoplasm before releasing it on the inward side, into your circulation.

That works fine for fresh live items of vegetation because they pass quickly to your intestine, still alive, and are easily recognised there – almost part of the taste process by which you decided to swallow them. That makes your gut reaction entirely friendly, precise and comfortable. The same is not true of protein or starch. Both have been cooked, and though eaten fresh (and tasting accordingly) have been in your stomach digesting for several hours since then. If any 'soul' is still attached, it may be quite different and certainly diminished by the time it reaches your intestine.

That is why your gut reaction to cooked food is initially hostile. The digestive leucocytosis is the result, long recognised by biologists but not completely understood until Bircher-Benner got to work on it. This defensive flare-up spoils the process of absorption, of course, and corresponds to chemical gastritis in your stomach. If it is the usual state of affairs it becomes chronic and deep-seated – an insidious step towards irritability or inflammatory disease.

If you eat raw, live food first, of course, this does not happen. More remarkably still, the cooked parts that follow in the same meal are welcomed equally well. That must represent a fairly recent adaptation in our 'soul' life, perhaps a few hundred millennia old. It certainly can't be explained by a mutant gene. And it offers a wonderfully simple way of nipping gut inflammation in the bud.

BLACK MARKET

There is always a villain in every story, and your intestine's is commonly known as 'leaky gut syndrome'.

Chemicals that you eat accidentally – whether pesticides, antiseptics, fluoride, artificial colouring, bleach or detergents – may encourage the skin of your mouth to ulcerate, but are generally resisted successfully all the way down through your stomach. They first register drastically on the delicate skin of your intestine. Whole clumps of skin cells can be destroyed or disabled, producing microscopic breeches in the lining. These bleed and inflame, trying to heal and often unable to because of continual exposure to the chemical damage. The discomfort, only dimly felt for itself, sets off stronger griping contractions in the muscle coat of the intestine, which are much more intrusive as the waxing and waning of colic.

The breeches have disastrous internal consequences. They are loopholes by which food material – let alone the chemicals that do the damage – can enter your body without being invested with your 'soul'. They stay themselves, circulating in you but unresponsive to your shaping influences. So your immune system recognises them, rather belatedly, as foreign, and reacts to cast them out. The result is generalised and uncomfortable – anything from vague aches and pains to something resembling 'flu. Your surface layers may inflame, provoked from within – resulting in asthma, sinusitis, catarrh or eczema, or any combination of them all.

A similar leak is created when the fungus *Candida albicans* gets out of hand, but that subject gets us a little ahead of ourselves.

THE SLIPPERY SLOPE

Your intestine is quite long – usually about ten metres or 30 feet. It is suspended loosely in a double fold of the skin that lines the back of your abdominal cavity, so that it can wriggle to its heart's content. Series of waves ripple along it, mashing and stirring the contents as well as pushing them along.

In the process, of course, the bulk of the contents diminishes as much of it is absorbed. This is despite the juices and mucus that may be added, some of which is waste and intended for excretion. The bile, for example, usually contains a little of the fat, cholesterol and fat-soluble material your body wants to get rid of.

So the character of the content changes progressively along the length of your intestine, from a loose rich jelly to a scantier, thicker, sewage sludge. It is highly coloured because of the pigments in the bile – yellow at first, then green and eventually brown.

The gradient of this change depends heavily on how much fibrous cellulose the meal contained. This is the chief agent that takes up moisture and swells into a jelly, stiffening the intestinal contents into a semi-solid. This not only protects the lining skin from too direct a contact with anything harmful it may contain, but it keeps the volume of the contents relatively large. So your intestine propels it onwards faster, to stop it ganging up anywhere.

The idea of a gradient works in two ways, then, but in opposite directions. If the character of the contents changes faster, through lack of fibrous content, the gradient of flow through the intestine is slower. If the contents change their character more slowly, stabilised by a high fibre content, the gradient of flow is much steeper.

If you are thirsty this contrast is accentuated. Your body absorbs more of the moisture in your food, to keep your own fluids at the right concentration. This dries out the contents of your intestine even more, further slowing their transit. This effect is far less drastic if your meal contained plenty of cellulose fibre, however, which is very reluctant to part with its moisture; so transit remains relatively quick.

Thus, the character of what arrives in your bowel varies enormously according to the kind of meal you ate, and what you drank. We shall look at its fate in the next chapter.

Chapter Seven: Profoundly Moving

Once you have eaten a meal, you lose control of its fate for the next part of its journey. How it will fare in your intestine and how fast it will reach your bowel are pre-ordained, and so is the way in which it will be treated in that sewage farm of your system, the caecum.

Of course I speak in general terms. You could exert yourself athletically, indulge in serious fairground aerobatics or give yourself an unpleasant shock, any of which could affect your digestion drastically. And the cumulative effect of all previous meals has a bearing too. Your first decent meal on top of a legacy of bad ones still cannot be dealt with properly. Even then, however, the next point at which you have any conscious influence is when and how you empty your bowel.

THE CAULDRON OF DISEASE

When your stomach swells to receive a meal, the previous one is shunted onwards as a whole, emptying most of its product into a large bag beyond. This bag is called the caecum, pronounced like Harry Secombe. A good meal arrives in your caecum just a few hours after you ate it, as a considerable quantity of loose featureless jelly – perhaps a litre or two, arriving in the course of 30–60 minutes. It is slightly alkaline or neutral in reaction, stripped of all obvious value and tainted with any undesirable chemistry you have either declined to absorb or actively excreted.

So if you manage things well your bowel receives an occasional surge of jelly from the intestine, not a steady liquid trickle. To the germs that have taken up permanent residence in your bowel, this is meat and drink. They thrive on cellulose, and in breaking that down release the small-chain starches, called oligosaccharides, contained in pockets within the cellulose structure. This is a great delicacy, which they turn into organic acids. So the colonies of germs multiply enormously, taking over the whole batch of material from the meal and acidifying it. The volume dwindles all the while as moisture is absorbed. Gentle churning motions of the caecum ensure that the entire batch ripens in a few hours more. This generates one or two kilograms of *acidophilus* germs per meal, in a healthy person on a perfect diet. Most of these die, giving their contents back to you. The rest go down the toilet, but a seed colony survives in the appendix – a hollow cave the shape and length of an earthworm, situated near the valve that separates the bowel from the intestine.

This valve, the ileo-caecal valve, is important because the caecum is a fermenting tank, with a leathery lining rather like that of the stomach. It therefore resists harm from the sewage farm it contains. But the tender lining of the ileum– the last part of the intestine – would not like it at all. If the valve opens by mistake, the seething backwash into the intestine severely upsets it. The lining itself easily inflames. Odours and excreta get absorbed through it unintentionally, making you unwell, paling your complexion and tainting your sweat and breath. Traditional Chinese doctors blame this for 'black rings under the eyes', but European medics don't seem to attach much significance to either leakage of the valve or the pasty complexion it causes. Too disgusting to dwell on, perhaps.

This misfortune is far more likely to happen if anything is wrong with what you eat. Scanty fibre content delays the meal residue and reduces its volume. There is not enough for the acidophilus germs to feed on, or even partly to fill the caecum, so the colony never really gets going. Instead of ripening promptly it dithers, drying out excessively. In the process its irritant contents become more concentrated and have more access to the lining of the caecum, irritating it despite its defences. This may trigger the valve to open inappropriately. More likely, it opens to release the next meal before the previous one has been discharged. Either way, upward leakage can take place into the defenceless intestine.

As by now you will imagine, that is not all. Most low-fibre diets also have a good deal of protein in them. Meat fibres from a large meal may well succeed in passing the entire intestine undigested – particularly if your stomach was not allowed time to get in the proper mood to do its job. Some of the germs in your caecum are wise to this. One is called *Escherichia coli* – the notorious *E. coli* that sometimes rampages lethally through hospitals and old people's homes. In a good, fibrous diet this germ is a harmless acidophilus, a positive contributor to the life of your caecum. Feed it too little cellulose but regular meat instead, however, and it changes its preference. It starts to digest muscle fibres, creating ammonia and all kinds of mayhem. Ammonia is strongly alkaline, which destroys the acidic climate created by and for the acidophilus germs – which by definition love acid and hate alkali. So the sewage farm is wrecked and becomes an *E. coli* enteritis instead.

That extreme is, thankfully, unusual. Lesser degrees of degradation are very common. It is rare now for the caecum to support more than a few ounces – perhaps 100 grams – of acidophilus germs, because there is too little food for them, and too much meat. Often that means the faeces cannot be properly formed: they are expelled as diarrhoea by an irritable caecum that will have none of it.

Otherwise, a host of different fermentations can take hold, easily overriding the weakened acidophilus colonies. Meat residues rot in the caecum because they have been retained too long – quite apart from whatever *E. coli* may do. That inflames the lining chronically, perhaps producing noxious diarrhoea. Offensive alkaline gases like ammonia also intoxicate the muscles of both the caecal bag and the ileo-caecal valve, contributing to the breakdown of their function. The caecum retains its contents far too long. Scanty residues produce only small desiccated nuggets like sheep droppings: too few to pass even daily. They mount up in a pile, the oldest and driest on top. Eventually the burden is great enough to provoke the strong bowel effort it takes to shift it outwards. In the worst cases, it can take up to a week for such faeces to be discharged – with great straining and discomfort. Even then, the bowel is seldom cleared completely.

THRUSH

One contributor to these upsets deserves a section all of its own. It is probably very common, a major cause of leaky gut syndrome and can make you ill and feeble for a very long time. Yet it is perfectly treatable, and must be tackled actively if you are ever to recover from it. To prevent or treat it you must first understand it, so here goes.

Carnivorous behaviour by *E. coli* creates alkali in the caecum. If you also – or alternatively – eat lots of bread, especially as meat sandwiches, undigested starch grains will penetrate into your intestine where you cannot do anything further with them. Apart from being irritant, like sand in your shoe, they encourage colonies to form of any fungus capable of surviving inside you, coping with alkalinity and living on these starch grains.

The most notorious of these is called *Candida albicans* – nicknamed thrush. The particular feature of this fungus is its ability to take two forms. Like most fungi capable of infesting your skin, it forms a system of rootlets and stems – a mycelium – which resembles a microscopic rhubarb patch, rooted in your skin. Most of these other fungi cannot get inside you, however, because the acid conditions of your stomach dissolve them away.

Thrush is different, because it can also form tiny cells, in the same way as bacteria, and survive in your intestine. Usually they live peacefully in small numbers in your mouth, and again in the lower intestine and bowel, not taking root and doing no harm However, if they are fed too well, or aided and abetted by *E. coli*, they can not only spread more widely but also change into a mycelium and take root in the delicate skin of your intestine.

This creates a fertile opportunity for black marketing. Anything absorbed by the fungus can, in principle, get past the intestinal skin layer without getting customs clearance. So, in addition to fermenting the starch in your meals to alcohol and passing that on to your circulation, it can inject you with all manner of other hostile fragments.

This condition is very debilitating, and completely undetectable outside of your body. The main symptom that gives it away is the outrageous amounts of wind you produce. The thrush behaves like a brewery, with carbon dioxide gas its most obvious product. This is responsible for uncomfortable bloating, and often blows off embarrassingly through one end or other; but may not do so if it leaks back into the intestine through a flabby ileo-caecal valve. The gas can dissolve back into your circulation and be breathed away instead through your lungs – though never fast enough to prevent bloating which starts after the first meal of every day and persists until bedtime. Doctors alert to this possibility can then check it by demonstrating the other brewery product – alcohol in your blood. This is proof positive: only thrush can change carbohydrate you have eaten into circulating alcohol.

I hesitate to get involved in needless controversy, but there's no ducking this one. *Candida* is a dirty word among doctors, who are only prepared to recognise its effects on the outside surfaces of the body – the vagina, the anal margin and sometimes the mouth. They are quite happy to treat these manifestations with appropriate medicines, for up to a week. Any symptoms that survive this remedy are then discredited in their eyes – even 'hysterical'.

Part of the reason for that is the exaggerated account of candidosis put about by some other writers on this subject. Their views seem to trace back ultimately to the work of Dr Orion Truss. He suggested that candidosis was a major epidemic, and advocated a diet devoid of any foods produced by, or capable of, fungal fermentation – which he considered would feed the candidosis condition.

I think this view is rather extreme. The diets people get on to in trying to follow Dr Truss's advice are draconian, leaving very few acceptable options. Indeed I would say almost none, since practically every natural food has the spores of its own fungal fermentation already living on its surface. One cannot survive a no-food diet for long.

But this is not the point. *Candida* is a very specific fungus problem, a rare exception – capable of travelling in the body as a seed or germ, but also capable of forming a 'vegetable' mycelium within the body once there. Not many fungi are capable of that – the *Aspergillus* species that produce farmer's lung is the other major threat of this kind, to human health. Other fungi are not tarred with this brush, and are relatively harmless to us.

The confusion is made worse because bread is so commonly eaten in such a way as to feed fungi rather than you. This is interpreted, quite wrongly, as sensitivity to wheat or to the yeast used to raise it (if you are so lucky) – leading to yet another major category of foods to exclude.

All this has discredited the entire account in medical eyes – and yet there really is a problem here. Once a fungus mycelium has become established inside you, it takes a lot more than a week's treatment to eradicate it. And I must say, despite my reservation about pharmaceuticals, that they do have a major part to play in this. There are some supplements and natural remedies that help to prevent recurrences and to prolong the benefit of pharmaceutical treatment after the prescribed course is completed, but few of them will produce a reliable cure speedily without such help. Certainly diet alone has not, in real time, produced a cure in any of the people that come to me. I have, on the contrary, more often had to rescue conscientious dieters from the near-starvation their efforts have produced.

There – I've said it. By all means write, if you must, and tell me about the latest expensive range of purely natural remedies for which you claim amazing results. Harangue me with the dire consequences of reliance on pharmaceuticals, if it makes you feel better – but I know all about that already, thank you. I will endure it all if a few more doctors will consider prescribing antifungal medicines for up to six weeks at a time, in those of their patients who report day-long bloating, or outrageous amounts of wind, in conjunction with either IBS or bizarre food-sensitivity symptoms. If they were unconvinced, perhaps they would at least organise a gut fermentation test in a few such cases. Whatever it takes, we need more doctors ready to treat these symptoms appropriately – which would set a lot of long-suffering people on the road to recovery much faster.

Having got that off my chest let's return to the main line of our journey.

THE FINAL TWIST

During the time a batch of healthy food is processed in your caecum, some nutrients and a lot of moisture are absorbed from the fermenting liquid into your circulation. The brew shrinks and gradually solidifies, churned by the mixing movement of the caecum's muscular wall. This motion acts like a potter's hands, forming the contents into a solid cylindrical shape, poised away from the caecal skin. By this time the risk of backwash to the intestine has passed, and the appendix has retained a sample of the culture in its own microclimate, with which to inoculate the next batch.

Once the fermentation and re-absorption of the batch is complete, your caecum contracts decisively to throw the faecal mass onward round the overhead loop of the bowel. The muscles of the colon are quite special, with stout strands along its length that act as drawstrings to shorten whole sections of the tube, like a concertina. So long as the contents are slippery and soft, and have successfully separated from the caecum in the kneading process, these extreme movements are nevertheless slick and comfortable. The mass passes through the remainder of the bowel in just a few seconds, usually without your being at all aware of it. This up-and-over section of the passage is necessary, or the caecum would brim over and spill its contents before they were ripe. But it is a clearway, not a parking lot. The faecal load should be free to pass down into the lower colon, on the left side of your abdomen just above the pelvis. The first you should know of it is an immediate signal – 'I want to go!' – when the mass arrives at the buffers, in the descending colon.

That is what you are aiming for. You should be emptying the remains of last night's meal the following morning – a transit time of about 12 hours. You should probably expect a smaller, softer, second action later in the day – particularly if your breakfast was substantial.

GO SLOW

In the First Movement I speculated that our ancestors, from the most remote up to at least mediaeval times, emptied their bowel several times daily – probably after each substantial meal. By the Napoleonic era, however, things were different – at least occasionally. 'Le petit caporal' himself was said to move his bowel only once every ten days or so, and then prodigiously. More reliable evidence from nineteenth-century surgeons, voiced by Arbuthnot Lane, was of ancient, turgid faeces bloating patients' bowels from stem to stern – their walls thickened, scarred and hardened by decades spent groaning under the burdens they carried. And since abdominal surgery was new, practitioners had never seen anything to suggest what might pass for healthy.

As late as the first half of the twentieth century, some writers of books on personal hygiene were circulating very mistaken views of normality. They include quaint drawings to show how far along the length of the bowel the meal would have reached by the second, third and fourth days after consumption – culminating in triumphant evacuation after anything up to a week. That is still grossly abnormal, however favourably it compares with Lane's patients! Evidence that this may even now be the rule, not the exception, will be found in many suburban loos – rows of books to pass the time during what is expected to be a protracted undertaking.

When did the slow-down occur? If Henry Fielding's *History of Tom Jones* can be believed, eighteenth-century innkeepers could provide large joints of meat accompanied by vegetables, and coarse bread. Huge meat meals were customary among the gentry by Regency times, usually without obvious penalty apart from gout and obesity. The bowels of the day must have managed to cope more or less with the vast throughput that resulted.

We can be confident of this because we know something of the history of that archetypal medical condition, acute appendicitis. The appendix is very susceptible to blockage by small hard faecal pellets, such as would occur in any bowel at a standstill. It can suppurate when colonies of *E. coli* get out of control. Both these conditions arise when movement through the bowel is drastically slowed. Until the late nineteenth century appendicitis was a rare disease, so the wholesale slow-down in bowel traffic must have begun towards its end – at about the time that refinement of flour became commonplace (Chapter Five). It appears that loss of the fibrous component in wholemeal bread was the calamity that brought overloaded bowels to a dead halt.

The tendency to such gross and stubborn sluggishness has eased a lot in recent decades. Appendicitis is on the wane as more people get the fibre message. But we are by no means out of the wood yet. Erratic bowel behaviour has taken over, swinging unpredictably between the extremes of total inertia and gross overactivity, according to the balance of opposed reactions from day to day. The non-nutrient chemicals that accompany modern meals – such as aluminium, fluoride, pharmaceuticals, detergent and pesticide – may irritate the bowel lining directly and disturb disastrously the germs in the bowels sewage farm, hurrying everything along painfully at first. If the damage to the local climate is extreme enough, however, the narcotic effects of the alkaline fumes, combined with a typical fibre consumption still much less than two centuries ago, can tip the balance the other way. From pangs of agony, the caecal muscle lapses into limp unconsciousnes – bringing everything to a crashing halt. Between these extremes we have sufficient explanation of the predicament you find yourself in – symptoms of both extremes, balanced uneasily on a knife edge and triggered unpredictably at the least twist or turn of fortune.

So how do you break the vicious circle – at the irresistible force, or the immovable object? You need the force, so you have to clear the obstacle. Constipation is still the key to your problem, despite all modern appearances. Let's see where you stand on that.

CONSTIPATION

Look at the questionnaire on p. 93. All the scoring answers in the box are indications that your intestinal transit time is too long, because there is not enough substance passing through to maintain the gradient from your mouth to your anus (Chapter Six). A steep gradient means vigorous activity all along your gut, with a brief transit time. Your faeces are therefore soft, featureless, moist, pliable and inoffensive and pass easily. Constipation is anything less than that.

Most people score at least 5 in this test. A regular daily bowel habit does not mean you are not constipated. Go by the consistency of what you pass. If it is dried out, it's been in your bowel too long. If it is made up of nuggets pressed together, or contains small pellets, that's bad news too. Each nugget or pellet

Are You Constipated?

Try this simple self-assessment.

Opposite each question tick the one box that most nearly applies to you.

After you have answered all the questions, score each answer in the larger box on the right.

Then add up your total score.

For interpretation, see the text.

Tick (value)

Do you empty your bowel?

More than twice daily	☐ (0)
Twice daily	☐ (1)
Once daily	☑ (2)
Less often	☑ (3) score: ☐

How long does it take?

Over five minutes	☐ (2)
1–5 minutes	☑ (1)
Seconds – a minute	☐ (0) score: ☐

Do you need to strain?

Yes, always	☒ (2)
Sometimes	☑ (1)
No	☐ (0) score: ☐

Is your stool

nuggets/pellets	☑ (3)
A stiff torpedo	☐ (2)
A soft 'snake'	☐ (1)
Looser than that?	☐ (0) score: ☐

Do you feel properly empty afterwards?

Yes	☐ (0)
Don't know	☐ (1)
No	☑ (2) score: ☐

Grand Total: ☐

is the result of one batch process in your caecum. They contained too little fibre to retain enough moisture to be any bigger or softer. It also means the emptying of your intestine is happening in more frequent dribbles – a feeble gradient.

If you recognise items in your faeces that you last ate days ago – tomato skins, beetroot, currants or seeds – then you have a traffic queue in your colon that should not be there. Each time your caecum empties, it adds one more nugget to the back of the queue. If they don't make it up to the 'hepatic flexure', they may fall back when the caecum relaxes and hang around in the bottom of the next charge. This is the way appendicitis starts – one of the small pellets gets into its opening and blocks it.

As the line of nuggets moves slowly across the up-and-over section ('transverse colon') they dry out and shrink even more, so that by the time they reach the head of the queue they probably don't even stick together. The give-away is a few pebbles at the beginning of the action, followed by a torpedo of compacted nuggets, progressively softer towards the back end – which will be blunted where it rested against the next torpedo, which is still in there.

If you pay attention to the sensations that arise from your abdomen, you will quickly realise you can feel when the caecum is filling up. If you poke it gently a little afterward – it's located in the right side of your abdomen, just above the hard bony rim of your pelvis – you will be aware how full it is. If it is sore, it has yet to recover from the irritating after-effects of previous meals.

The pain of constipation arises because the bowel contents are not easily shifted by the large concertina movements of the bowel muscle. So they strengthen, and still only nudge the mass a fraction of the distance it should have gone. They continue like that indefinitely, in colicky waves, working almost in vain on a queue that barely moves. Your impulse to 'go' becomes indistinct, lost in the background noise of regular pangs.

STING IN THE TAIL

Every inch of the bowel has to put up with this, day after day. Inflammation and irritability can be taken for granted, the norm.

Pressure from the bowel's own muscles during periods of constipation, and irritant contact of its lining with abnormal stools – whether rock hard or liquid – have accumulative consequences.

Piles are the earliest to appear. These are swollen skin and blood vessels around the margin of your anus, brought about by the need to strain in an effort to get rid of faeces that are too dry to empty just from bowel contractions. Piles can become as large as hen's eggs and are usually sore, though seldom really painful. They often bleed because they burst under the pressure within them.

Or the lining of the anus may crack, torn open by the hard surface of a dry turd scratching it. The tear starts on the inside margin, hurting sharply, and bleeds a little. The nubbins of skin torn away by this remains attached, of course, forming a handle by which each successive turd can make a contribution. The tear therefore extends a little each time, hurting and bleeding some more; but the older part of the tear heals up gradually too. By the time the tear has reached the outer margin of the anus – a total distance of about three cm (one inch) – it can heal completely, leaving only the tag of skin dangling on the outside, to mark where that fissure has been. You can have a whole series of them of course – even several at once – until you stop the cause.

Some effects take longer to form. Constant high pressure inside the colon is like the air pressure inside a bicycle wheel. If there is a weak spot in the tyre, the inner tube pouts through it and may burst. That is exactly what happens over the years in the bowel of a habitually constipated person. The lining skin of the bowel (the inner tube) needs blood and nerve supplies, which reach it by passing through small portholes in the muscle layer (or tyre) of the bowel. When the pressure builds up inside, the skin is supported by the muscle everywhere except these portholes, which bulge slightly. Over time these holes widen under pressure, and eventually a pouch of the inner skin pouts through, covered only by the fibrous coat outside the muscle layer.

These pouches are 'diverticula' – just a Latin translation. The condition of having several diverticula is called diverticulosis. If the diverticula contain foul material they can fester and become abscesses, which may burst and produce an abdominal disaster.

They are entirely bad news, therefore. Fortunately most diverti-cula remain too small for that and diverticulitis – inflammation – is uncommon; abscesses are almost rare.

The end stage of the process is a bowel that is not only punctuated with diverticula but heavily laden, bloated, torn, stiffened and fibrous – the sort of condition Victorian surgeons were so often presented with.

Cancer occurs mainly in those parts of the bowel that are most subject to prolonged contact with irritant contents – the caecum at one end and rectum at the other, the last part of the bowel before the anus. It is surprising that these structures take so long to give in to the disgusting conditions they have to put up with. Nevertheless, I have known youngsters of around 40 get bowel cancers, if they ate enough meaty food. What is more, they have survived very well after treatment, provided they improved their diets radically enough.

That's enough of an exceedingly unsavoury subject. It is time to spell out exactly how to avoid, or remedy, any such thing.

GETTING IT RIGHT

If your predominant symptom is irritable diarrhoea, you need to get all the inputs corrected including prescribed and over-the-counter medicines, where possible – and you should start notic-ing improvement within a few days. Chapters Eight and Nine give more detailed assistance. You may well need to feed yourself with live cultures of the germs your caecum needs to work properly, and you will certainly benefit from a short period on the Cleansing Diet detailed in Chapter Ten. You may also for a time be glad of remedies containing herbs such as comfrey, aloe, mint, chamomile, or homoeopathic medicines such as Arsenicum album, to help you reduce your reliance on pharma-ceuticals and to soothe the irritable lining of your bowel whilst awaiting radical cure (see pages 122–125). You should probably take a bit of advice about these, for which the WellDesk premium line (page 177) may prove helpful.

Somewhere along the line the irritation should wane, and you may swing the other way into a constipation phase. It is not likely to become anything like so dire as I am about to assume, but I must cater for the most severe and protracted kind of stoppage. Again, you may care to call the WellDesk help-line to work out a measured response to your particular need.

The rules for getting your bowel back on line are given in the box on pages 98–99.

I am not a great advocate of self-administered enemas, though I am satisfied they can usually be handled safely if need be. The problem with them is that they tend to become a habit, and that should not be necessary. The theory is that hard, dry faeces get stuck permanently on the bowel lining, rather like plaster on a brick wall, and cannot otherwise be cleared. Sometimes this may be true, but in that case I would advise the temporary attentions of a professional colonic therapist, preferably with a nursing background (see Useful Addresses), rather than self-help. If you decide to carry on despite this warning, do at least get some assistance from the Cytoplan Help-line (see Useful Addresses).

If the result of all this is disappointing, there are three other conditions you need to consider – probably with professional help.

In the first place, your thyroid gland may have slowed down a little, reducing your body heat and general metabolic power. This produces a stubborn form of constipation, often at an early stage in the onset of the condition. Unfortunately, the blood tests usually done to detect this are not as reliable as most doctors think, and you may need outside help from a specialist doctor more familiar with the problem. Full details are available on page 102.

Secondly, your stomach may no longer be capable of producing enough acid for protein digestion. For some reason that I cannot explain, this too can produce a difficult constipation. As this is part of the picture in pernicious anaemia, if you know already that you suffer from this – as well as constipation – an acid-releasing supplement with protein meals is wise. Betaine hydrochloride may be available to you on medical prescription and is offered by several nutritional catalogues. You may find, however, that vinaigrette (see page 128) on the protein dish is just as effective, tastier and more economical. So long as you do not get heartburn symptoms, you are not having too much.

Thirdly, your 'soul' may be implicated. If you have acquired a relevant miasm (Chapter Four), you can clean up your body as

- **Avoid or minimise (phol)codeine-based pain- and cough-remedies, and all antispasmodic medicines** which have the worst record of constipating side effects.
- **Drink half a litre of water before each meal**, to activate the gastro-colic reflex and to reduce dehydration, which you would otherwise try to correct by drying out your faeces too much.
- **Whenever you sense a need to go, go!** Don't wait, even a few minutes, if you can help it. That signal means you have propulsive movement in your bowel ready to help, for the moment; it won't last.
- **Squat properly** – not easy on a British toilet. Your legs should be well bent up and apart at the hip, and your body leant forward a little, to straighten the lower bowel and make movements easier. A 10cm wooden stool to stand on, on the floor in front of the loo, makes this much easier for some people. The continental squat-hole may not appeal aesthetically, but it is bio-logical!
- **Try never to strain,** which is where piles, anal fissures and varicose veins come from.
- **Intensify your bowel's own effort** by breathing with your diaphragm. 'Belly-breathing' is detailed in the box on

much as you like – it will still follow the wrong pattern set by the miasm. You need to consult a psionic medical practitioner about removing the miasms that affect you (contact details are on page 176).

SUCCESS

The road to recovery from constipation (with or without irritability) may be a little prolonged – several weeks would be usual – and you need some idea how to judge when you have arrived.

Don't be put off by much more obvious signs of bowel activity – temporary bloating, wind, noises, brief colicky pangs. These are sure signs that your bowel has aroused itself from sluggishness, the gradient has steepened – things are on the

page 127. This will put nervous energy into your bowel, and you'll start to feel it contracting.

- **Don't be satisfied with one brittle turd.** Wait a little longer, still breathing as above. With luck you may pass the next one along, and even the next, thereby reducing the backlog. Give yourself up to five minutes total for this – no more.
- **Use the body-wrap** (see page 126) to soothe your gut and intensify its housekeeping between bowel actions.
- **Consider natural stimulants – NOT bulk laxatives.** Syrup of figs will intensify the contractions of your bowel muscle, even before the syrup has passed through your system. Fresh coffee has the same effect but instant is not so effective. Bran, flax seed (linseed), and other bulk agents only work as they pass through your gut so you have to empty your bowel properly first, to make way for them to get through.
- **Splash your backside well with cold water,** after you have completed your session. Pat dry with a towel rather than paper. The only use for paper is to remove fragments of faeces that are still attached round your anal margin, before you wash. Install a bidet, if you have room for one: otherwise extend the cold tap on your bath with a short length of plastic garden hose, or an old rubber shower adaptor.

move. But your bowel is out of practice, its muscles are unfit and hung-over, and it will be a few weeks before everything settles into a rhythm that you cease to be aware of. It also takes a month or two for a healthy bowel and intestinal lining to grow through from scratch, without which you cannot settle into maximum efficiency.

The texture of your bowel products is the prime indication of success. They will be soft, featureless, bulky, capable of coiling in the pan without fracture. They should pass easily without straining, be inoffensive, and heavy enough to sink in water. You may recognise in them fragments of what you ate yesterday. There will be a feeling of satisfaction once you have emptied your entire bowel properly, which should quite quickly be every time. To maintain that, you have only to keep faithfully to the diet and meal habits this book has been about. You may for a time, or in some circumstances, need help from fresh linseed (up to one tablespoonful daily, well chewed before swallowing, prior to any substantial meal) but try to keep off the syrup of figs.

Cereal bran is fine, consumed along with the remainder of a whole cereal food (check products in Chapter Nine, and page 125). It should never be eaten dry off a spoon – despite Cleave's Naval prescriptions (Chapter Two) – because it may not moisten evenly and ends up in sticky lumps which may actually worsen constipation. If you feel you need a concentrated form of bran, try Brose (see p. 125).

Piles need longer to settle completely. The keys to curing them are absolutely no straining, ever; and lashings of cold water after each action. You may do well afterwards to put on an appropriate ointment, or insert a suitable suppository, to reduce the inflammation between actions and make more rapid progress. Painful piles need ice as first aid, because they have clotted: your doctor can sometimes help with special ointment for this situation.

Anal fissures eventually reach the outside and form a skin-tag that will dangle there for ever. By then the fissure will have healed – it takes several weeks, as a rule. Your new healthy bowel habit will prevent any more.

You may have general setbacks. Try not to be dismayed by how easily they can happen, even after months of normality. Some of the situations that cause them can be prevented, however.

The worst scenario occurs when you have to travel. Any substantial journey, whether by road, rail or air, can completely shut down your bowel for that day. I suppose it may be a helpful reaction in a way – you certainly don't want to be caught short urgently in mid air.

There are two tricks for dealing with this. The first is to see whether you can get your bowel to empty before you set out. This is safely possible, without straining, once you are used to breathing its muscles into life. The second dodge is to drink plenty of water during the journey. Most travellers tend to dry out – air travel appears to be the worst for this – and need consciously to drink regularly. Coffee and tea are counter-productive and best left out altogether: they hurry the water out through your kidneys, so the dehydration persists. Remember to abide by the rules for good digestion throughout the day, too, so that you get back to normal rhythm quickly next day.

And that is the story – all you really need to know. The Third Movement adds a lot of detail you may find useful, but you are already equipped to work most of it out from first principles for yourself. However, you'll want to get it absolutely right, rather than waste recovery time over a simple mistake, so flip through to check the details that appeal to you. And keep the WellDesk number handy (see Useful Addresses) – in case of urgency.

Slow Metabolism

Metabolism is chemical work within the body. The rate is determined largely by the activity of the thyroid gland, which in turn is regulated by the pituitary gland at the base of the brain. Metabolic rate can go up during a fever, which is part of your general defences against infection, for example. It can go up and down fractionally with your state of arousal – psyched up for a sporting event on the one hand, or curled up against the cold on the other. I suspect that people with ancestors from the far north of the world are capable of partial hibernation, so that in winter they metabolise more slowly, and get up more reluctantly, than in the summer.

Doctors are not generally aware of any of this because we have changed the method by which we measure metabolism. We used, until about the 1950s, to measure it directly – long-winded and expensive, but accurate. Now we rely on tests of the level of thyroid hormones in the blood, which is easier and cheap but can be misleading. It turns out that the best substitute for the fill-blown test of metabolic rate is your basal body temperature, measured at rest after a good night's rest in bed.[1]

Your basal temperature may be depressed for a few other reasons, besides thyroid insufficiency. If you are on a strict weight reduction diet, or ever had jaundice severely, your basal temperature may be low and your thyroid function normal. If you are taking 'beta-blocking' medicines for angina or blood pressure control, this lowers your metabolism and basal temperature and thyroid treatment will not restore it to normal. If none of these apply, a basal temperature regularly below 36.6 degrees C or 97.8 degrees F may indicate that you are thyroid-deficient, or inclined to hibernate. This is happening insidiously to more people, and at younger ages, than formerly. A possible reason is the rising consumption of fluorides (Chapter Five).

If your thyroid is under-active, for whatever reason, this will be a very stubborn cause of constipation. It may have other important implications, too. To put matters right you will need specialised help, and should contact Good HealthKeeping (a membership organisation) or WellDesk (available to anybody) for further guidance (see Useful Addresses).

[1] BARNES, B.O. (1976) *Solved: The Riddle of Heart Attacks*, Fort Collins, Colorado: Robinson Press.

Third Movement
The Secrets of Success

Chapter Eight: The Natural Course of Events

Life is punctuated by memorable events, which, in the case of my wife and me, are often associated with memorable meals. They range from a gigantic hors d'oeuvre at the late lamented Stage Door bar in Norwich, to an impromptu meal of an exceedingly fresh trout, and a lucky success with the Hollandaise sauce we threw together for it.

Part of the delight of such occasions is their relative rarity. None would have been half so pleasurable if repeated the following day. The trick is to make equally special the everyday meals that fill the long spaces between banquets. Your health and digestive constitution are founded entirely on these routine offerings, so they must combine many virtues. Freshness, nutritive value variety, interest and safely low pollutant content you can arrange by the way you shop. Digestibility and flavour are modulated by how you cook and prepare. But the health and comfort of your intestine, and its fitness to face the next meal after this one, are down to the sequence and arrangement of the meal.

This is the only part of your catering that you can safely entrust to routine. Indeed, being the routine is the secret of its success. People sometimes notice straight away the benefit of a good meal arrangement, the first time they do it. But nobody gets more than a fraction of the benefit available until they have followed the system regularly for several weeks.

The reason is very simple. Each correctly arranged meal sets you up in a slightly better condition to deal with the next, so your digestion becomes progressively more and more efficient. Your gut gets a chance to heal. This illustrates a basic axiom of health, that the more you have the more you will receive. It may not sound fair, but it is the way nature has always worked and political correctness will not change it.

However, even the thought-police cannot criticise what I am about to tell you. The secret of good digestion, and therefore of a healthy gut, is available to everyone regardless of social or economic position. Whatever you eat will go down more comfortably, and nourish you better, if you choose and arrange it well. That is priceless – but entirely free of charge. If it were possible to package, brand and sell it, I'm sure we'd all have heard of it long before now.

DRINK, OR SHRINK

Human beings are not designed to graze. It doesn't work in the rain forest, so don't try in the urban jungle. If you get peckish during the working day, don't eat: drink instead. Air conditioning, travel, brisk movement and hard labour all dry you out, but this doesn't register as it should. Somehow or other we've got our wires crossed. In the early stages of thirst we feel hungry instead, and only start to feel dry when we're thoroughly parched.

I do not understand how the switch came about, but I'm quite certain it's a mistake. On the hoof, your mood is all wrong for eating. If you go for confectionery or biscuits, you set the wrong digestive juices flowing and upset your stomach. Your appetite for the next meal is spoilt and your stomach will not be ready for it. Whereas if you drink, your stomach gets rinsed clean and has nothing else to do but let the liquid through. Your body fluid gets topped up before the first hint of drought, and any surplus spills harmlessly through your kidneys.

It does matter what you choose to drink, of course. Many mid-morning beverages have drawbacks. The worst snag is the xanthine derivatives, a class of chemicals that includes caffeine, theophylline and theobromine (as well as nicotine). These are the defining ingredients in tea, coffee, cocoa and cola, all of them stimulating and therefore popular. However, they stimulate your kidneys as well as your mental processes, so that the fluid comes out almost as fast as it goes in.

I had this brought home to me during an expedition to Egypt, 36 years ago. We were motoring home along the long North African coastal road, a journey of nearly two weeks. Our routine was porridge and coffee before an eight o'clock start. The five-hour driving session until lunchtime was invariably punctuated by a pause for bladder relief at about ten a.m. One morning, however, the stove blew out before we could make the coffee: we grumbled, and drank water instead. The drive that followed was uninterrupted – none of us even thought about relief before we stopped for lunch.

These customary hot drinks are better than eating, but they don't rehydrate you and are rather habit-forming. A strong brew is also apt to irritate your stomach. Try the Mediterranean habit of drinking a long glass of water, then a short shot of good coffee. I'm not so keen on tea because I once fell victim to its fluoride content (Chapter Five) and guess that some other people do too, without knowing it. Even good tea is more-ish, whereas one's appetite for decent coffee is more easily satisfied. I keep off drinking-chocolate because of all the sugar it contains. Proper cocoa is bitter, as satisfying as good coffee and more nourishing, but harder to come by and tricky to prepare.

As to alcoholic drinks, they get your kidneys working and lower your blood sugar, which accounts for its use to stimulate appetite. Mixers and spirits are far more likely to cause gut problems than real ale or good wine. Most mixers are now chemically concocted. Spirits are alcohol distilled away from a fermented brew, leaving almost everything else behind. Because you need other food items to deal safely with alcohol, a tot of whisky or gin is in effect a negative meal. It creates additional demands in your liver that must be satisfied from other food sources.

Proper beer or wine, on the other hand, is still virtually the whole brew and contains a wide variety of other food elements, either made by the yeast or added to ensure its survival. It is a meal in itself. This lightens the pressure on your liver to some extent. Besides, the far deeper quality of taste tends to satisfy you sooner, and to wane after a few glasses, so the temptation to keep on drinking is far less. None of this can be claimed for brews that are fortified, or treated chemically to shorten the fermentation process, clear cloudiness or alter the taste. Alcohol is dangerous during the day. The evening is a different matter.

Proper fruit juice is a legitimate drink, but when you are thirsty it is possible to drink enough to lower your blood sugar, which is counterproductive; so always dilute it at least 50 per cent with water. And if you toil hard enough to need a solid snack, you can follow up your drink with a piece of fruit. A ripe banana is the most digestible and sustaining, but an apple or pear is better if you are getting near a mealtime, since these will not spoil your appetite.

That leaves pure water as your best bet for quick breaks. This is a subject in itself but the bottom line is simple: the purer, the better. Put tap-water through a filter jug, at least, to remove chlorine and any traces of organic chemicals. But fluoride and hardness minerals are undesirable as well, so that a still or reverse osmosis unit is an investment worth serious consideration. Distilled water is in my opinion too pure to be the perfect answer, and the running costs are on the high side. I recommend reverse osmosis as the best all-round solution, yielding very pure water at about 1 penny per litre (five pence to write off your initial investment within the first year).

If you prefer the more expensive option of bottled water, choose only those which advertise their mineral content and reject anything with a total dissolved solid figure (TDS) greater than about 30–70 mg/litre. Also beware of a fluoride content above about 0.2 mg/litre or parts per million (ppm). If the label does not list either of these contents, leave it on the shelf.

Hard water is reputed to protect your heart, but that's a dishonest spin on the scientific evidence. If your food is magnesium-deficient, the magnesium in hard water helps to stop one form of heart attack. The proper answer for that is magnesium-rich food, in which case the magnesium in water is not just irrelevant – it becomes actively harmful, according to the evidence. Calcium in water is unreservedly bad news. Water minerals are not food, so they cannot nourish your bones; but they can, and do, harden arteries and contribute to stones in your kidney and gall-bladder.

If you decide to go for bottled water it will be hard to avoid plastic. Plastics are like glass – not really solid at all. They are usually made of polymers – large jigsaws made of many copies of one basic piece, a simple chemical. But jigsaws always have edges that tend to fray, allowing small amounts of the basic chemical to be released. This is responsible for the characteristic smell around fresh plastics, and for traces of pollution dissolved in the contents. Glass is much better, since it's far more stable and the basic ingredient (silica, i.e. sand) is pretty harmless. But since so few bottled waters are available packed in glass, you may have to go for the larger (5 litre) plastic bottles – less of the water is in contact with plastic. And start saving towards a permanent reverse osmosis unit under your kitchen sink.

If your work is physical or in hot conditions, you will perspire salt as well as water. Without salt you cannot keep water in your body, so replace that as well. You can season your food with up to a teaspoonful of sea salt daily in total, or you could use vegetable bouillon as a salty, savoury hot drink.

Doctors have overdone the message to limit salt. We are rather helpless to prevent high blood pressure and its effects, so we exaggerate the advice we give. Salt – sodium – is essential in the body. Your blood contains a third of one per cent and your whole body around 100 grams (over three ounces). What you lose you must replace, or else your body fluid will shrink – regardless of what you drink.

Soft drinks – including lemonade and colas – are a mixed blessing. Most of them now bear very little resemblance to the original recipes, relying heavily on artificial flavourings and sweeteners. Many of them now contain added caffeine: colas always did. The 'diet' versions usually contain aspartame, which can be converted to formaldehyde in the body and is suspected of causing nerve damage – so avoid these, pending a verdict. Ingredients like these are apt to trigger inappropriate acid release in your stomach, and to encourage the wrong bowel germs. I strongly recommend you keep right off all of them.

As to 'alco-pop' and sport drinks – after all these remarks, need you ask?

MATTERS OF COURSE

A three-course meal is probably no longer the routine habit on weekdays, even in the best regulated households. Most of us are content with a substantial meal on one plate only. Nevertheless, that plate almost certainly contains the makings of three separate courses.

You have to remember that your gut is a single tube, with no sidings or passing-places. We have established that different sections of that tube are specialised for different kinds of digestion. It follows that, for the best possible result, you should eat every meal in the same order as the arrangement of specialist sections along your intestine. That way everything can be digested at the same time, each in its own proper place.

We have dealt at length with the value of drinking first of all. Watery fluids pass straight through the stomach, in little time at all. They are absorbed from the intestine in a few minutes more, again without digestive effort.

The same applies if the fluid is fresh juice, with an added bonus. Enough of the fruit's 'soul' persists to switch off the digestive leucocytosis. That, you remember, is the angry inflammatory reaction provoked accidentally in the skin of your intestine by cooked and dead food. Accident it may be, but it unsettles your digestion and you are better off without it. This is why the juice of a freshly squeezed orange finds favour as an apéritif. We drink preserved fruit juice in vain: it may be a pleasant prelude, but has no digestive benefit.

What fresh juice does well, whole fresh fruit and vegetation does better. It takes a little longer to reach your intestine because you take time to chew it, and swallow it in smaller mouthfuls. But it still does not linger in the stomach, so long as it is not heavily dressed with oil or mayonnaise. Fat slows the emptying of the stomach, which adds substance and stay to a quick salad meal but is not wise as a prelude to richer fare.

After the live vegetation comes any that is cooked. By now the leucocytosis is no longer a risk and digestion is very like the preceding raw food, and in the same place.

At this point it pays to put down the cutlery and wait a moment, even if the entire meal is on one plate. Don't embark on anything more until your stomach is comfortably empty again. A sense of fullness at this stage probably means you have eaten the vegetables too fast, so you need to steady yourself in any case. But the main reason is to create a hiatus between one form of digestive task and the next.

If your meal includes anything very savoury or rich in protein – meat, poultry, fish, hard cheese, lentils or solid soya products – this is the item to tackle next. Take your time, chew each small mouthful well, and appreciate the flavour. The outlet of your stomach will promptly close, sealing off the intestine and its vegetable contents. Mucus and acid juices will start to flow. The protein and juice will assemble, mouthful by mouthful, in the protective mucus envelope in your lower stomach, which will enlarge rapidly to accommodate it.

This stage in the meal is absolutely not to be hasty or thoughtless. It calls for concentration in your mind as well as your stomach. Savour the moment. A sophisticated creature has been reared with care, and somebody has invested yet more care in preparing it for the table, all of which deserves careful appreciation on your part. Believe me, this is what it takes to digest that protein perfectly. Without you achieve that, all manner of mischief can arise later on.

You are under no obligation to eat every scrap of this, the richest part of the meal and hardest to digest. Once you sense you have had sufficient, stop and rest a moment. If your appetite returns, continue by all means: if not, you have had enough of that.

Do not be tempted to eat potatoes – less still bread – while there is protein left that you intend to eat. A little extra vegetable is not so disruptive, and an occasional sip of wine may even help. Starch of any kind is incompatible with your present objective: it comes later. You need that protein course isolated.

Hay, whom I introduced in Chapter Two, would have you stop the meal at this point. He maintained, quite rightly, that the acid climate required for the digestion of meat is so completely incompatible with the neutrality called for to digest starch, that they were better segregated into entirely separate meals. In a country where meat is eaten on a massive scale, that is excellent advice. Even in Europe, up to the nineteenth century, meat was consumed in great quantity by the well heeled – often accompanied by bread or pastry. By now, however, portions have become smaller and the range of choice has narrowed. There are now somewhere between 3 and 5 million vegetarians in Britain, a massive growth in recent decades.

In these circumstances it is not the size of the meat portion that matters so much as the contrasting quality of digestion it requires. That can safely be confined in the lower half of the stomach, leaving the upper available for starchy food if you need it.

Puddings became customary as an inexpensive combination of fat and flour to fill the hungriest members of the family, who worked the hardest and spent the most energy. The entire household had a share of the more precious parts of the meal – the vegetables and meat – after which those who were still hungry could have as much pudding as they needed.

Whether this eating habit prompted the digestive adaptation or vice versa, we shall never know. The fact remains that we are well equipped to cope with a meal served in that way. The pudding or bread, mixed with saliva, forms up in a semi-solid mass in the upper stomach, isolated from the protein below by a muscular tightening around its 'waist'. Only in that way can you get the benefit of cereal foods at all, because the starch they contain must be broken down by saliva into simpler sugars before these can be further digested and absorbed in the intestine.

Potatoes came later, and complicate the situation. The starch in potato is much easier to digest, though it still requires some attention from salivary enzymes. However it usually gets classi-fied with vegetables now, rather than as a separate course, and eaten alongside meat. There are many recipes in which potatoes are used to thicken stews and casseroles, and I have to admit that these are not obviously indigestible. If you have no digestive problem or intestinal disease you may well get away with food of this kind; but if you know you have trouble, it is far wiser not to try. You need to be as kind as possible to your intestine, so that it can serve your nourishment and at the same time heal up soundly. In the most acute situations it is better not to eat rich protein food at all, as we shall see. Even when things are coming under control, it is foolish to take obvious risks.

SERIAL CEREAL

If you have been accustomed to think of starchy food – espe-cially cereals – as a light snack, think again. Fresh fruit is a light snack: cereals are serious business.

We saw in Chapter Three that foods from seeds of the grass family are our most recent digestive accomplishment. It is really important to set their breakdown off on the right foot, and to give it adequate time for completion. That means reserving the top half of the stomach, especially the fundus, to receive the starch exclusively and with similar attentiveness to that we should give meat. Starch that does not break down sufficiently in your stomach will not break down further in your intestine, and not nourish you at all. But it can still irritate the crypts of your pyloric antrum and your intestine, and set off excessive mucus production. It can still feed the wrong germs and fungi in your intestine and bowel, ruining the function of the sewage farm you rely on to sanitise your bowel contents. So get it right.

- Rule One: only eat cereals wholemeal. These have sufficient fibre to become gloopy when you have chewed them sufficiently. In this semi-solid state you have a chance not only of retaining them successfully in your upper stomach for the required length of time, but of creating the right not-quite-liquid texture to the contents of your gut, right through its length. Cereal fibre is particularly valuable but seed fibre in general – especially linseed (also known as flax-seed) – has this property.
- Rule Two: choose organic, or at least unsprayed cereals. This is for the purely practical reason that cereals are usually sprayed with herbicide very shortly before harvest, to kill a weed called black grass that tends otherwise to grow in the stubble. The heat of a stubble fire once helped control weeds but burning stubble is now illegal, so farmers rely even more on chemical sprays. The spray residue cannot be washed off and is therefore trapped in wholemeal flour and eaten. We have no idea how much this upsets the gut in otherwise healthy people but I know several people who can manage organic wholemeal very nicely, yet react against flour that isn't.
- Rule Three: eat cereals alone, and as dry as possible. They need to absorb all the saliva they can get: milk or spread that gets there first dilutes the digestive effort that will be available. And of course a bowl of milk with cornflakes floating in

it stands no chance at all of staying remotely solid in your stomach.

There are ways of beating this necessity, by taking the rule to extremes. Toasting a cereal thoroughly splits open some of the starch grains, releasing more loose ends of sugar for digestive enzymes to work on simultaneously, speeding up the process. Biscuits – literally, twice cooked – take the principle even further by creating a brittle product with even more thoroughly crumbled starch grains. The more modern crispbreads benefit from the same advantage. Even bread that has gone stale is more digestible than a freshly cooked loaf. All these items should be eaten dry.

Breakfast cereals have been corrupted very much as desserts have. They are a far abstraction from the muesli and porridge that inspired them. If you want to do the job properly then use the recipes nearby.

- Rule Four: ditch sugar, confectionery and desserts. So few of us now toil sufficiently to need filling with energy, we hardly need consider pudding and pastry. Custard made with powder bears no relation at all to the confection of eggs and milk that originally bore that name: it is sweet, loaded with refined cornflour and deadly to taste-buds and digestion. O.K., it evokes memories of school dinner in anyone old enough; but that's about it.

    More intricate confections of fruit, sugar, ice-cream and chocolate may be delicious, but to anyone with digestive problems they simply represent danger. If you want chocolate, just eat that – bitter, no milk, at least 70 per cent cocoa. It's available in most supermarkets and quite a few High Street shops, it's good and it's actually rather nourishing. At the end of a savoury meal is also a sensible time to eat it.

- Rule Five: neither eat nor drink anything else at all for several hours after eating starchy food. You need that starch in the uppermost compartment of your stomach for that length of time, if you are to survive the meal without problems. Anything else – even a tiny cup of coffee or tea – ruins your chances.

And that is all. I have been telling you all along how simple the message is. If you are not impressed, you haven't yet tried it properly. The devil is in the detail, of course, so let's look at that.

BREAKFAST

This is an important meal which you should not usually neglect. It is better to eat a hearty breakfast next morning rather than a large dinner late the previous night.

There are two basic patterns to the European breakfast – Continental and 'Full English', though the Irish, Welsh and Scots know just as well, if not better, how to breakfast fully. North Americans adapted the polyglot habits the original settlers brought with them. Their main independent contribution is excessive portions. I find the Arab breakfast habit particularly appealing, and suspect that was the ultimate source of breakfast preferences all round the Mediterranean margin and throughout the Middle East – whoever may claim them.

Continental
- Satisfy your thirst first. Drink a long glass of pure water; unfiltered tap-water improves with a drop or two of lemon juice. Go on to a smaller glass of freshly squeezed juice, if it appeals to you. (Some people love milk, but I don't recommend it.) I admit to a liking for good black coffee, and sit comfortably over a cup or two at that stage before eating anything. You can of course substitute any variety of hot brew (no milk or sugar).
- Eat any fruit next – preferably a piece or two fresh, or a fresh salad, but a stewed compote also serves.
- (If you intend to attack the cold cuts of cheese or meat, this is the time. Don't eat the bread of an open sandwich yet – eat only the toppings first. Never mind the looks.)
- Finally – the cereals (croissants), rolls or bread of your choice. (No fatty spreads and only low-sugar preserves). Toast or bake bread as lightly as you can get away with – burnt cereals do you no favours.

If you are trying to control your weight, omit the items in brackets: details are in Chapter Ten.

'Full English'

- Again, drink first: water, juice and hot beverage according to your thirst and preference (without milk or sugar).
- Fresh fruit or a bowl of fruit salad, prunes or fruit compote fit nicely here.
- Kippers or mixed grill settle splendidly at this stage. Cook each item well, but not too crisply. We usually overcook fish grossly, which is a terrible waste and bad for your digestion. Kippers take only two to three minutes each side under a hot grill. (Avoid fried bread, sausage, black pudding, potatoes, hash browns and ordinary baked beans.)
- (Toast and spreads come last – if you truly need them).

If you are trying to control your weight, omit the items in brackets: details are in Chapter Ten.

Arab

- Drink first, much as in other traditions. Always drink water with or before your coffee. Avoid the sugar if you get the choice.
- Any fruit or peppers on offer come here, dressed and seasoned by all means. Yoghurt is a good accompaniment to this course.
- If you care for cheese, fish or fellafel (meat balls), segregate them to this stage.
- Now settle to your choice of pitta-bread, humus, olive oil and digestive herbs.
  Ah!

Personally, I would not spoil an Arab breakfast with thoughts of weight control. Arabs are not famously fat. Savour the moment, eat only what you really have appetite for, and walk it off later.

My usual breakfast? I take my time over a well made organic black coffee (half of it water-processed decaffeinated), America-style. Then a few rounds of home-made organic wholemeal toast with sugarless marmalade or fruit conserve. We buy the wheat as grain and mill it at home, fresh for each batch of bread.

If I am travelling I treat myself to the full Anglo-Celtic breakfast. I easily gain weight so I drop all the items in brackets.

Unless I am anywhere near the Middle East. . . .

MIDDAY

In the best of all worlds you would eat your main meal at midday. The French have that exactly right. Alas, few can manage this before retirement, so you have two main options: lunch sparingly, or breakfast (or brunch) substantially and skip lunch altogether.

Get in the mood with a drink, by all means. At midday try fruit or tomato juice. If you are thirsty, drink plenty of water. It's not good to eat when you are dry because your stomach cannot make sufficient digestive juice, or create it at the right strength. If you drink later in the meal you not only upset the composition of the digesting mix: you probably wash it out of its appointed place in the stomach, to arrive prematurely in your intestine, not yet ripe for further digestion there. So do almost all your lunchtime drinking before you start to eat.

If you know you have a digestive or gut problem, do not arrange business over meals. By all means get to know people over lunch and do your business with them morning or afternoon, but make a clear break between the two activities. Switch off your mobile phone, and on no account open your palm pilot or laptop, until the meal is over.

If your meal-break is short, for whatever reason, tailor your ambition to the time available. Only attempt what you can complete without rushing. That usually means confining yourself to one course. You can manage a piece or two of fruit, at least. Organic, chemical- and GM-free items are obviously to be preferred, and are becoming easier to find. They will go on getting easier – and less expensive – provided you keep on asking for them.

In any case, sandwiches, filled rolls and baguettes are definitely out.

- Drink plenty in any case. The same rules apply as for breakfast: decent water first, then perhaps fresh juice. In some city centre bars you can now get juices fresh and substantial enough to replace lunch altogether – an excellent plan.
- Soup is an intermediate option but keep it simple – carrot, celery, leak and potato, minestrone, onion, tomato. Or straight fish soup such as clam chowder. Avoid 'wet casseroles' – meat and vegetable mixtures – which are too much of a digestive challenge. (Leave the roll until last).
- Alternatively, have a fresh salad of vegetables and fruit. It's best to avoid meaty components and pasta, so select carefully from a buffet. By all means dress with mayonnaise for added substance.
- You can go the whole hog – soup followed by salad (but postpone any bread until the very last).

Omit items in brackets if you are trying to control your weight.

My own workday habit is literally to forget lunch altogether. I have regular hot drinks of vegetable bouillon and the occasional coffee (always fresh) through the day. Occasionally if we are toiling hard at the weekend we'll have a piece of cheese at lunchtime, or suitable leftovers from the previous night.

EVENING MEAL

For the best, your evening meal should usually be sophisticated but light. For the multitudes who end their working day by relaxing over this meal, and may not have eaten at all before that, here's a menu for survival.

- Sit and muse over a watery drink. You are probably quite thirsty, though you may not know it. Avoid sweet soft drinks. If you prefer beer, try watering it a little to extend it: alcohol keens the appetite, but enough full-strength beer to slake your thirst may dull your taste. In general, satisfy your thirst on water before embarking on alcohol in any form.
- A small dressed fresh salad of live fruits or vegetables – tomato, grated raw carrot, seed-sprouts. Any live yoghurt you intend to eat should accompany that.

- Dish up your main course on one plate by all means, but eat any cooked vegetables next. That excludes potatoes, pie-crust or croûte, flan-case, rice and batter, which come in the starchy category. Unless you toil long and hard in the course of your work, you don't need their wonderfully fattening qualities anyway.

  Cook leafy vegetables only as long as it takes for them to wilt and go vividly green. That happens suddenly, at the moment when the cellulose cells of the leaves burst open and give access to their contents. If you prolong it, you spill out those contents into the vegetable water and devalue the leaves. Steaming and wokking are the safest methods.

- After a brief pause, eat the protein part of the main meal next, on its own. Take your time. That could be the filling of a quiche, pie or croûte – complete with sauce. Cheese, nuts, beans and soya dishes – tofu, textured vegetable protein or TVP – qualify alongside meat of any kind, fish, game and poultry. Do not char meat – cook it just enough.

- If you fancy a piece of cheese as a final course, omit all starchy items until after you've had it. A plain hard oat biscuit or crispbread would go down well then, but not before.

- Finish with as much of the starchy vegetables or pastry as you dare. On the whole, unless you really have worked hard physically during the day, you are better off leaving out starchy food altogether at your evening meal. If your evening includes sport, you will not want to burden yourself beforehand, and afterwards you will have no opportunity to burn it off.

That's how a lot of people put weight on – storing up starchy food eaten at night, which they had no immediate use for. It's much better to eat well at breakfast, generating the energy right there when you want it, during the toil to follow.

SNACKS AND SUPPER

The best food at any other time is water, to slake the thirst you may not realise you have. If you are genuinely weakening at the

Checklist for Good Digestion

	Task	Detail page	Tick
GENERAL	Consider psionic medicine, to get rid of miasms	41	☐
	Check your metabolism	102	☐
	Check your aluminium exposure	64	☐
	Check your fluoride exposure	65	☐
	Check your fluid (and salt) intake	106	☐
	Check your stomach acid	97	☐
	Check your medicines	61, 98	☐
BUYING	Organic	52–55	☐
	Fresh	36–38	☐
	Whole	50	☐
	Seasonal	55	☐
	Local, known sources		☐
	Consider live yoghurt	26	☐
	Remember to minimise aluminium	64	☐
COOKING	Separate protein from starch in all recipes	109-112	☐
	Remember to minimise aluminium	64	☐

EATING	*General*		
	Drink first – no spirits	106	☐
	Business-free zone	117	☐
	Nothing sweet on empty stomach	75	☐
	Chew well, savour reflectively	110	☐
	Courses		
	1. Live fruit/vegetables	79	☐
	2. Cooked fruit/vegetables	81, 110	☐
	3. Protein	110	☐
	4. Starch	112	☐
DIGEST IT	Pause before next action		☐
WASH UP	– whether by hand or machine –		
	Hot water with no detergent **or** Minimum detergent and generous rinse	66	☐
BOWEL?	Any signal – act promptly!	90, 98	☐
	Breathing	127	☐
	Take time (up to 5 minutes)	99	☐
	Don't ever strain	100	☐
	Wash with cold water (e.g. bidet)	99	☐
	Consider linseed	99	☐

knees, try to rely on a piece of fresh fruit only. The energy is light, accessible and very digestible. Sweet biscuits, snack bars and confectionery are out – you risk too much (Chapter Six).

In general it's better not to snack in the evening or eat before going to bed, but that's a rule honoured more in breach than obedience. Nuts, pumpkin or sunflower seeds and pine kernels are the most nutritious. If you tend to be constipated, it makes sense to nibble fresh linseeds, dried figs or a compote of stewed figs and prunes.

If you find you settle better to sleep after a small meal, the best choices are a banana, hot milk or a cereal with milk. All these tend to improve the sleep that follows. The least risky is a really ripe banana – black spots on the outside, softening in places inside. This is predigestion rather than rot, and quite safe to eat so long as it tastes good.

NATURAL GUT REMEDIES

Aloe Vera
Unless your bowel is very loose, this is the best single herb for soothing an irritable bowel. Half way between a cactus and an onion, its fleshy leaves are filled with a spongy gel. This was originally extracted by slitting the leaves along their length and stripping the pulp, rather like shelling peas. Now the whole leaf is macerated and pressed, which unfortunately mixes into the pulp the undesirable, irritant sap from the plant's veins. The best brands remove this again by absorption onto activated charcoal, so that the gel is reliably non-irritant.

Drink a small wineglass (50ml) of the neat gel twice daily on an empty stomach, until you begin to improve. Dilute the concentrated versions (e.g. nine parts of water to one of a 10:1 concentrate). You can reduce the dose as you improve.

Angelica leaf
Do not confuse this with the crystallised stem, used in cakes and confectionery. Angelica leaf is a powerful liver tonic, and can be taken as a herbal tea.

Chamomile

A soothing flower tea you can use to help calm an over-active bowel, perhaps as a substitute for Asian tea or coffee. Available in most health shops. See the box on Herbal Teas for details of preparation.

Cider vinegar

See Chapter Nine.

Comfrey leaf

This fleshy herb is native to Britain and can often be found growing wild in the corners of gardens or meadows. Apart from its content of vegetable protein and vitamin B12, and its gardening merits, comfrey has healing properties – it speeds up the activity of white blood cells to four times normal, without apparent ill-effects. Overall, it accelerates the whole healing process by about 30 per cent, which is useful in healing your gut more securely. Take as fresh leaves in wholemeal sandwiches, or as a tea – one rounded dessertspoonful per pint, per day.

It came in for a bad press during the 1980s when eight comfrey alkaloids were reported capable of liver damage. However, comfrey consumption would have to be inconceivably huge, and articles in both the main British medical journals exonerated comfrey leaves and stems as safe. The root has more alkaloids and was withdrawn from medicinal use – a great loss to sufferers of mouth ulcers.

Grapefruit seed extract

Once your doctor has given you as much antifungal antibiotic as he is prepared to prescribe for suppression of thrush (Chapter Six), this is a good thing to follow up with. It is available least expensively as drops, which are rather bitter, and as capsules. You will find many products in health shops or can obtain it by mail from WellDesk or Good HealthKeeping.

Intestinal Herb Formula

Many herbal mixtures are available that soothe bowel irritability but I particularly recommend one formulated by a practitioner from the Balkans, Nigel Vukovich. It relieves the symptoms of irritable bowel syndrome, dramatically but safely, while you organise your cure. Take 0–3 tablets before the next meal according to your symptoms since the previous one. Available by mail order in packs of 200 from Good HealthKeeping (see Useful Addresses).

Lemon Barley Water
This bears only a nominal resemblance to commercial cordial. For its convalescent benefits while soothing your upset bowel you must make it yourself:

- Cover 2oz (50gm) organic pearled or pot barley with pure water in a pan and bring it slowly to the boil, stirring to prevent clumping or sticking. If the remaining moisture looks dirty, strain it off: otherwise retain.
- Add a further pint (500ml) of freshly boiled pure water and stir for 30–60 seconds before straining into a jug and allowing to cool. (NB brew too long, and your water will gel on cooling.)
- Add lemon juice, to taste.

Linseed
Also known as flax or hemp (distinct from Indian hemp or marihuana), the seeds of this plant are the best natural bulk lubricant remedy for constipation and an excellent source for vegetarians of essential fatty acids of the omega-3 and omega-6 series. The oil goes rancid very easily, so I strongly recommend you eat the seeds, chewing them to obtain the oil. 1–2 tablespoonsful daily are a sensible amount. Available in bulk and inexpensively from health shops or by post from Cytoplan Ltd (see Useful Addresses).

Peppermint
A readily available herb you can use in cooking, as a herbal tea, or even in emergency as a sweet. An excellent way to calm a digestive disturbance – hence their popularity after a complex main meal. I recommend you buy the loose herb and drink the hot brew – see Herb Teas on page 128.

Propolis
This is the special antiseptic wax bees produce to use when constructing their hive. It maintains the most germ-free environment found in nature, and has been shown to help heal an

ulcerated or inflamed gut. I do not trust watery 'concentrates', as most of propolis does not dissolve in water. Extracts in general are less effective than the whole material. A reliable product is obtainable by post from WellDesk or Good HealthKeeping (see Useful Addresses).

BRAN AND BROSE

This usually refers to wheat bran by default, but oat and rice bran are also commercially available – though less effective at regulating constipation. All come from the outermost skin of the cereal seed and are valued for the quality and quantity of the indigestible fibre they contain. Loss of this from the diet at the end of the nineteenth century, when most bread became 'white', is probably responsible for the rise of constipation and appendicitis.

Bran is at its best raw and fresh, when it will absorb moisture rapidly and become a stiff jelly. It is best eaten very moist and mixed with other cereal elements as part of a wholemeal recipe, when there is no danger of adverse effect. If bran is eaten pure and dry it can produce sticky lumps in the gut, which have a paradoxical constipating effect – they can stick to the lining of the bowel and slow the transit of other food.

Buy your bran loose, and insist on organic material. Cereal crops are often sprayed late, just before harvest, and most of any residue will be in the bran.

Brose is the safest and most effective way to eat bran. Here is the recipe:

- Mix 1 cup of coarse raw organic oatmeal with 2 cups of raw broad (i.e. flaky) organic bran and 1 handful of organic raisins – all readily available from health shops.
- Sprinkle this mixture into 4 cups of boiling water, and stand for 10–15 minutes, during which time the ingredients swell and soften. If you possess a slow cooker, you can place it on a very low heat overnight – the result is much more solid, even a cake, depending on the freshness of the ingredients.

This amount will probably last you several days, but don't stint yourself!

Body Pack

This is a simple application of hydrotherapy that you can use perfectly safely to ease IBS. It will not mask anything serious, though it may prevent or even cure an early case of appendicitis.

Prepare a cloth of worn cotton or linen – an old sheet or a couple of tea towels – that will go round your body once, from the bottom of your ribs to your pelvis. You will need enough safety-pins to fasten the overlap every few centimetres. And you must soak it well in cold water, then wring it as dry as you can, before you get in the bath.

Have a fairly long hot bath or shower, during which you may like to massage your belly slowly and gently, in clockwise circles. You can direct the shower nozzle at your belly and move it in circles instead, if that is easier.

Get out and dry off, then wrap the cold cloth once round your tummy tightly, using the safety-pins. The entire cloth should be firmly applied to your skin. If water squeezes out, you have applied it too wet. Put your warmest woollen jumper on over this.

The initial reaction is a cold shock of course, but that quickly converts to a tingling glow. Touch the skin under the margin of the cloth – it should feel hot to your finger. If so, it's working – leave it on for two hours. You can dress up normally, or go to bed, with the pack still on.

BREATHING

Breathing properly is an essential part of overcoming any bowel problem.

The diaphragm is a thin dome of muscle stretched across your body between the bottoms of your ribs, the dome projecting upwards under your heart and lungs. Two thirds of your lung space lies in the few centimetres just above your diaphragm, and remains almost unused, unless you breathe in chiefly by drawing your diaphragm downwards. This inevitably pushes your guts forward, making a prominent belly profile – so what?

To learn how, place one hand on your ribs under your armpit and another on your navel, and breathe in. I guarantee your ribs will move. You have to learn to put the effort into raising your navel, and then to still your ribs completely. You should be able to breathe perfectly well with your ribs encased in concrete.

Once you have the elementary skill, start to exercise it regularly. Breathe in deeply and slowly with your diaphragm, to a count of 5; then hold your breath in for 5 more; then exhale gently for a further 5 before commencing the next inbreath – a three-phase cycle. Hold your breath in by the effort of your diaphragm, not in your throat – every other muscle around your belly should relax too. Keep this up for a minimum of 10 breaths on each occasion. When you have the knack extent the count to 7 – just over 3 minutes for 10 breaths.

This will clear your head and calm your mood whenever you do it. Nervous energy is drawn down from your head into your abdomen, where it is used only for good purposes – healing and house-keeping. The Body Pack (see page 126) can be used to amplify the result still further.

Herbal Teas

The chief problem with Asian teas for IBS sufferers is their fluoride and tannin content. No tea from south-east Asia is free of fluoride, since it is richly represented in the soil, and the tea bush thrives on it. Consequently the better the tea, the more the fluoride – green tea particularly.

Rooibosch (Red Bush) tea from South Africa is, however, very similar and contains far less fluoride. It is obtainable in many health shops and a few supermarkets.

Another alternative is cider vinegar and honey (see p. 135). The ingredients are easily available organically in supermarkets and health shops, and it is very easy to make.

Herbal teas are quite a different type of drink, but can be combined in brews with similar strength of taste. They can be chosen to assist your digestion and soothe your gut – try peppermint, chamomile, angelica leaf and ginger as ingredients.

Use fresh leaves where possible, 1 teaspoonful per breakfast cup, or 2 teaspoonfuls of dried leaves not more than a year old. Chop and crush them, and add water that is not quite boiling. Allow to draw for ten minutes. You only need strain off the leaves if they persist in floating after you have stirred the brew.

Vinaigrette

- Put in a blender or mixing bowl 25 ml (1 fl oz) of organic cider or wine vinegar – you can make up some of the volume with organic lemon juice if you prefer.
- Add a little pepper, salt and mustard and blend them together.
- Slowly add 50 ml (2 fl oz) of cool olive, wheatgerm or sunflower oil whilst blending continually.
  This way the oil will emulsify and the sauce will thicken and stabilise. Prepare freshly for each meal.

Chapter Nine: An A-Z of Food Choices

The list that follows is not exhaustive. It covers a wide range of food types, dealing with them in general rather than specifically. Having adopted alphabetical order, I have listed some items in several places.

This is a personal list, which flouts various official nutritional guidelines wherever I think fit.

You should find here a point of reference for every type of food you buy, and sufficiently detailed comment to enable you to make a reliable judgement of the value and safety of each specific brand you may consider buying. You will also see when in the day, and where in the meal, to eat it.

Item	Comment
APPLE	Unless the fruit are certified Organic or Biodynamic, the skin is liable to harbour spray residues which are likely to penetrate a millimetre or so into the underlying flesh. Washing in water removes dirt, but not spray residue – peeling fairly thickly is wasteful, but much more effective and worthwhile if you have a problem to deal with.
	A good choice for a snack between meals, since it combines moisture with a little starchy nourishment. First course of a substantial meal.
	Stewed apples and life yoghurt, exclusively for two days, is a boring but effective way to dislodge the wrong germs growing in the caecum, and get acidophilus types restarted (see Second Movement). See also Cider Vinegar.
APRICOT	Fresh apricots have a short season in Britain and are imported, so liable to be quite heavily sprayed. Dried apricots are usually treated with sulphur dioxide to preserve their orange colour, which may upset you even after cooking (which drives off most of the sulphur). Do not nibble bright yellow dried apricots – the sulphur dioxide will almost certainly unsettle your digestion.
	Unsulphured apricots are a dark brown colour but far safer for nibbling.
ARTICHOKE, GLOBE	An excellent, delicate edible flower. Often used pickled, or steamed with a buttery dip, as a first course to a main meal.
ARTICHOKE, JERUSALEM	A root vegetable, or more accurately a tuber (like potato). These are starchy, and usually need lengthy cooking because of their fibre content. Quite hard to digest. Best avoided if you know you have a digestive problem.
ASPARAGUS	A premium crop with a short season, and a suspiciously rapid increase in availability over recent years. Both suggest caution: try to find organic options, as spraying is very likely unless certified otherwise.
	A shoot, so suitable for a salad or as first course to a main meal. Usually served steamed with a buttery sauce or dip. The tips are tender and easier to digest, the stems become increasingly fibrous the further from the tip you venture to bite.
AUBERGINE	An oily fruit related to tomatoes and peppers, in Greek cuisine the basis of moussaka. Being a substantial and tasty item, it can be used as the centrepiece of a

vegetarian main course. Imported from various Mediterranean countries and almost certainly sprayed, unless certified otherwise.

AVOCADO

The fleshy fruit of a large tree, grown in the Middle East and Southern Africa. Organic options are available and well worth the extra, since this is an intensively sprayed crop otherwise – though the thick outer skin provides some protection.

In the process of ripening the flesh 'turns' at a certain point, becoming cheesy and digestible where previously it had been rubbery and tough. You can choose by feel (no need to poke hard) and buy early to await ripening, or choose ripe ones to eat today. The former is chancy since they may begin to rot while you wait.

Cut the fruit open, peel off the skin and slice finely; or eat out the flesh with a spoon, like a boiled egg. Either way, goes well with an oil and vinegar dressing. A fine centrepiece for a salad or seafood dish.

BACON

This is pork part-cured (i.e. preserved) in a modern process involving nitrates, which, if anything, adds to the digestive challenge. To be eaten gently fried, grilled or baked, and better not charred or too crisp. Very much a meat course, not to be eaten in haste.

BAKED BEANS

Several generations of otherwise poorly nourished children have survived by courtesy of tinned baked beans, probably the best protein source they ever got. However, the tomato sauce contains a surprising amount of sugar and beans are famously indigestible. This is because of their rich combination of protein and starch – generally the starch digestion goes wrong and produces significant gas.

It's better to use fresh or dried whole beans, see below.

BANANA

Although these palm fruit are often sprayed with insecticide, most of it stays on the outer skin so the edible part is kept clean. Indigestible when green, the condition in which they are usually imported, they turn yellow during the voyage and become more and more digestible as they soften thereafter. The translucent softening is self-digestion rather than rot, so take advantage of the bargain batches, unloaded cheaply at fruit stalls before they liquefy completely! The actual rot is a firm, bitter blackness attacking the edible flesh: don't be daunted by blackening of the skin.

Probably the best convalescent food. If you intend

to eat one that is still firm and white, mash it and let it
stand for a while to make it more digestible.

**BEANS, FRESH
DRIED**

Beans are a rich combination of protein and starch
which is inherently indigestible. This is worse with
dried beans, which go starchy as they mature. Rather
than simply soak and cook them, it is far better to
sprout them first for a few days, until a shoot has
grown along the length of the bean inside its skin. By
that time the starch has been digested to sugar again,
and the beans may be eaten much more safely, raw or
cooked. (Sprouting also loosens the skins of red beans,
which are usually cooked for hours to reduce their
mild toxicity. Wash out the skins and you can eat even
these raw.)

Fresh green beans – including broad beans – are
much less rich and can be thought of as vegetables,
despite their protein content. Taken young enough
they are quite delicious and digestible raw, as a first
course. (also see soya)

BEER

If you can't afford to buy beer in glass bottles, brew
your own at home. Share one bottle between two and
add another third of good water – you'll not notice any
loss of flavour.

BERRY

These fruits have intense flavour and make good
conserves (see jam). They are a bit overpowering
alone, and are usually mixed with apples in fruit
salads, puddings and pies. Not a good idea after an
elaborate main course, but a fruit pie can successfully
follow a plain dish or salad.

BISCUIT

This very hot form of baking cracks open the starch
grains in the flour, making them more digestible than
they are in bread or raw cereal. However, sweet
biscuits are really confectionery and not suitable to be
eaten into an empty stomach. Savoury oat biscuits
serve just as well and are a much safer snack, though
ripe bananas are better still.

A savoury organic wholemeal biscuit or crispbread
is suitable after cheese, as a small meal or the last item
in a more substantial one. Rye and wheat crispbreads
will be excellent options once they are reliably
available as organic. Until so specified, they come
second.

BOVRIL™

see spread

BRAN

Raw bran may be bought on its own, but it is never
wise to eat it that way. It takes up moisture avidly,
producing a firm jelly of sticky lumps that can make
constipation worse. Dispersed through another cereal
the benefit remains and the danger is dispelled. Far

better, however, to eat a wholemeal cereal in the first place – in which case you'll not need added bran for long. Toasted bran flakes of any brand are poor value for money. Toasting largely destroys the moisture absorbency of the bran – the very property for which you are taking it.

BREAD
Wholemeal organic bread is usually available now, and you should not settle for less. Granary bread is not wholemeal but can be made with stained refined flour. White sliced bread, packed in plastic bags, is usually made by the Chorleywood process from refined flour that will support more moisture and air – there is very little substance or nourishment in it. Try squeezing a slice – it will consolidate into quite a small cube. Beware of sandwiches. Never follow bread with anything other than more bread. Eat it dry (with or without spread) and chew it well.

BURGER
A flat cake of ground meat could contain anything. Don't eat any you have not made yourself from good, safe ingredients. Cook them through, but don't char them. In any case do not serve meat or cheese in a bun.

BUTTER
Whilst in principle butter is far better and more flavoursome than vegetable margarine, it usually contains pesticide residues the cow has excreted in her milk. These dissolve preferentially in the cream, from which butter is made. Organic butter is therefore a great treat and far safer. Its relative rarity is a good discipline – you are forced to be sparing with it. (See also Mayonnaise)

CABBAGE
The inner heart of a cabbage may be tender enough to eat raw but the outer leaves are often bitter and always too tough to be digestible without steaming. They are cooked at the moment they go limp and a vivid green, simultaneously: this signifies that the cellulose skin has been burst and its contents are now accessible. Take them off the heat immediately, drain and serve. The cooking water is a valuable drink, provided it tastes pleasant.

CAKE
This should be classed with confectionery, never eaten on empty stomach and only then by thin or seriously hungry people. The combination of eggs, flour and fat tends to be indigestible and fattening.

CARROT
Beware the perfectly formed carrot, free of all blemish. Carrots hoard chemicals, and one insects have not dared to nibble may be loaded. Freshly grated organic carrots, however, make a quick and excellent raw

salad to start a meal, with or without an oil and vinegar dressing.

CAULIFLOWER

Beware large, perfect heads of cauliflower. They are difficult to grow like this without intensive feeding and protection. If smaller organic items are available you will find them more flavoursome and much easier on your gut.

They seldom need much cooking and make an excellent raw item, with or without a dip, to start your main meal.

CELERY

This savoury stem is not, in my view, very valuable as food. Its principal virtues are crispness and moisture, and a very low calorie count for slimmers. It also contains psoralen and oxalic acid (mostly in the older leaves), two irritant and undesirable substances. It is a viable alternative to biscuits as an accompaniment for cheese, and I have to admit that braising brings out a pleasing flavour.

CEREALS, BOXED

I am deeply suspicious of any cereal packed in a rectangular cardboard box, and the more elaborate they are the deeper my distrust. Flashing labels declaring added protein, vitamins or iron only make me despair that what rightfully belonged there was ever removed in the first place. You realise by now that the replacement falls far short of the original.

You are better off choosing ordinary organic porridge oats, usually available in plastic bags from health shops. The best of the boxed varieties is shredded wheat, the best-known brand of which is wholemeal and contains absolutely nothing else. It does not claim to be organic, however, and will surge forward to first equal on the day it does.

Use only as much milk as you must, aiming for a solid crumb structure – not flotsam. Don't add sugar – raisins, sliced banana or chopped dates serve far better, if you must. You may safely follow with bread or toast, but nothing else.

CHEESE

Like all dairy produce, cheese concentrates any pesticides the cow has excreted in her milk. These gravitate to the fat fraction, however, so low-fat cheese is safer. However, it never tastes nearly so good, so I prefer to spend more on a decently made organic cheese and eat it more seldom. It is a sustaining nibble between meals, and a very acceptable protein course in a more substantial one, provided you do not react to any pollutants it contains. You may get away with a scanty grating of mature cheese toasted on to the top of vegetable dishes – quality without the quantity.

CHICKEN Mass-production of chickens is, in my opinion, a pretty disgusting business, and the product hardly tastes of anything. Treat yourself to a free-range organic specimen occasionally, and leave the rest alone. You'll have no difficulty detecting the difference in cooking quality and flavour.

CHIPS, SEE POTATO

CHOCOLATE The substance called chocolate in England is largely composed of sugar. The Swiss and Dutch do it better – their bitterest chocolate may contain up to 75 per cent of cocoa solids. This is actually very good food, rich in minerals and protected from any sprays by the pod in which the beans grow. You can get it at a very reasonable price in almost any confectioner, supermarket or grocer's shop. Best eaten alone, between meals.

CIDER VINEGAR This apple-juice conserve is a time-honoured remedy. Apples are good all-round sources of nutrient minerals, in their most accessible and storable form: the concentration of each is low, but regular daily consumption means they accumulate usefully in your body. Only buy organically grown.

If your stomach is failing to make enough acid, cider vinegar is sufficiently sour to help you digest protein food – see vinaigrette. Combined in equal quantities with good honey in hot water to taste, it makes an excellent substitute for tea or coffee.

CONFECTIONERY Avoid it. Console yourself with a little bitter black Swiss chocolate occasionally.

CORDIAL Fruit-flavoured syrups, for dilution as watery drinks, invariably contain a list of chemical ingredients that are a minefield for anyone with an irritable digestion. The syrup in even the best of them is not good news. Go instead for fresh juice – even the heat-treated stuff in cartons – and dilute it with three parts of water. You won't miss cordial for long.

CORN (ON THE COB) A sweet, starchy seed you had best omit from complex meals if you have active digestive trouble. A roast or boiled cob goes down well with butter as a small meal on its own, though.

COURGETTE The best value of the marrow family, in my opinion. Sliced and sweated a little in butter or oil, it's a wonderful vegetable that shows off the superiority of the organic item. Easy to overcook, but usually excellent as your raw first course.

CRAB A seasonal delicacy and a wonderful treat, so far as I am concerned. Avoid manufactured 'crab sticks', they're not nearly so tasty. Very much the protein centrepiece of a main course salad.

CRACKERS

If by this you mean white puffed squares of biscuit, you'd be crackers to eat them. Maybe that's how they got their name. Wholemeal crispbreads are much better, though far from perfect.

CREAM

The dodgiest dairy item of all, since it concentrates the worst pollutants that a cow dumps in her milk. Try to avoid it. I've never seen organic cream, though I expect it's available.

CRISPBREAD, SEE BISCUIT

CRISPS

Genuine, plain potato crisps deserve an honourable mention, despite their content of overheated fat that may irritate your gut. You may get away with these as an accompaniment to cocktails, though olives would be safer. The exotic flavours are artificial, or course, and if you're wise you'll leave all crisp look-alikes alone. It's easier if you don't have the first one.

CUCUMBER

Conventionally grown items often taste faintly of dishwater and fishmeal, and have very few virtues. Organic ones are firmer, more substantial and do possess a subtle flavour of their own. You may draw your own conclusions. The latter are suitable for your raw first course.

CUSTARD

Originally custard was a dessert confection based on eggs and milk. The version based on tins of coloured cornflour bears very little resemblance to the original, and has none of its few virtues. Learn to live without it.

DATES

Sweet as they are, dates are a far more wholesome substitute for sugar in virtually any context – on cereals, in fruit salads or as a snack on their own. They are best eaten fresh rather than dried, and can be softened by cooking. Try to avoid the dessert trays that seem to be coated with syrup of some kind. Most health shops offer them unadulterated.

DESSERT

Whereas puddings used to make some sort of digestive sense, our modern dessert is an irrelevant vestige. Learn to live without cartons bearing this label. Their ingredients – principally sugar and fat – leave a lot to be desired, and they complicate the digestibility of a complex meal.

DUCK

Farmed duck has all the disadvantages of farmed chicken, but wild duck is something else – free range, and virtually organic. It is worth learning to pluck them, to be able to take occasional advantage of the game-dealer's offerings. You'll not want it often, which is as it should be.

EGG

Never buy anything but free-range – if you've seen inside an intensive poultry-house you'll know why, but the flavour is also far more rewarding and the colour of the yolk probably genuine. If ever you see them for sale at a smallholding you pass during a country visit, buy them – they're probably all-but organic.

FIG

Fresh figs are delicious but probably sprayed for transit. Dried figs may not be. They are the best natural aid I know to strengthen bowel contraction, and you can easily nibble your way through too many. A stewed fruit compote including them, apricots and prunes would be gentler, and could form the first or (after fresh fruit juice) second course of your breakfast.

FISH

This is very old food for humans, and far the best value of all meats. We generally get it stale and overcook it – it seldom needs much more than warming through to tenderise it into delicate flakes. Don't poach it in lots of water, and don't grill for more than a couple of minutes each side. Rick Stein heats thick cod steaks in olive oil to the temperature his finger just cannot stand, and in a few minutes off the heat it is done.

Fresh fish is firm in texture, with bold eyes, bright scales and no unpleasant smell. Don't be afraid to buy it smoked but ask for it without colouring – more producers are now catering for that.

FLOUR, CORN

If you use this to thicken soups and sauces, you clearly don't worry about your weight. This is the staple cereal in central America and parts of Africa, but is not so nourishing as wheat. Unless you particularly like Mexican food, it offers no particular advantage. It is not a safe alternative if you are allergic to wheat.

FLOUR, WHEAT

This is the staple food of western civilisation, drastically devalued when we began to refine it wholesale, then to spray the crop before harvest. Wholemeal from organically produced grain is now mandatory for people with gut problems. There's already a lot of it available and the supply is rapidly increasing.

Eaten as bread and plain bakery only at the end of meals, it gives very little trouble. As thickener in sauces for protein dishes, it is chancier.

FROZEN FOOD

Choose this rather than tinned, but choose fresh rather than either. There is some degradation of the food in preparation for freezing, and a lot more when you defrost. Having said which, a few frozen berries or runner beans are quite a tonic in February or March. Just don't live entirely out of the freezer and microwave.

FRUIT, DRIED

These are a fair substitute for confectionery, but best soaked overnight or stewed to soften them. Many are sulphured to preserve their colour, and are very indigestible unless soaked well. For nibbling purposes, only choose unsulphured versions. Avoid products treated with oil or syrup.

FRUIT, FRESH

All items are very basic food for humans, the ideal alternative to confectionery. Learn to love the items we grow in this country, and have a good go at them when in season. Exotic varieties have less reliable provenance and their spraying is less carefully regulated. Ideal items for your first course at any meal, or on their own as a snack between meals.

FRUIT, TINNED

These are best left on the shelf. Most contain syrup, and few bear much resemblance to the fresh item.

GAME

If you can't live without your meat, then the game-dealer is your friend. Wild rabbit, pheasant, partridge, pigeon, hare, duck and venison may be expensive but they are invaluable as clean sources of healthy, virtually free-range meat. They are one of the advantages of living in the country, but fresh game may be had in most cities, at a price. Always requires careful eating, on its own, as the protein course of a main meal: never rush it.

GARLIC

Some loathe it, but I love it. It is almost never served on its own but may accompany many salads and protein dishes with great profit. Fresh garlic has great medicinal virtues, particularly as an aid to keeping your body tubes and tissues clean internally. Garlic oil features in Chapter Ten, Cleansing Diet, item 10.

GINGER

Mainly used as a spice in hot recipes, it is also very digestive – hence the popularity of crystallised root ginger as an after-dinner treat. Not to be consumed in quantity, even so, if you have gut problems.

GOOSE

Sometimes available wild, but usually farmed. Their meat contains a lot of fat, much of which can be lost by roasting or on a grill. Choose free-range and organically grown.

GRAPE

Fresh grapes are vulnerable to rot in transit, so are always heavily sprayed. This is a pity, because they are excellent sources of minerals and very cleansing. If you cannot get organic grapes, use organic raisins instead – much easier to find.

GRAVADLAX

This is salmon that has been cured without cooking or

smoking. Traditionally done by burying the fish, the process has been modernised using sugar and herbs. It's a delicious alternative to smoked salmon, and about as digestible. A protein course, obviously.

GREEN
VEGETABLES

These are available fresh in season virtually all year. Boring they may be, but valuable too. Their cultivation need not be so intensive (except Brussels sprouts and cauliflower), so less spray is involved. Organic sources usually have good provenance.

Best steamed or wok-fried, just to the point of wilting. Not suitable for the raw first course but can follow it immediately.

HAM

Pork, more thoroughly cured than bacon, still with nitrates. Needs no further cooking and seems more digestible than bacon, but still rather a challenge. The protein course, to be eaten alone or with fresh mustard. Renounce ham sandwiches totally.

HERBS

These are edible plants used in small quantities chiefly for their flavour or medicinal properties. They are always better fresh than dried, so grow your favourites in pots. Renew your stores of dried herbs annually, only buying what you can use within 12 months. Mint, onion, chamomile, fennel, garlic, mustard, parsley, angelica and ginger all have good digestive properties. Useful as garnishes to meat dishes.

Aloe, angelica, arrowroot, ginger, slippery elm, and liquorice are used medicinally to aid gut problems. Comfrey leaf is useful to accelerate a healing process, after ulceration for example.

HONEY

This may cover a multitude of sins, even if obtained direct from a beekeeper. Honey extracted the day after the bees were fed with sugar is still only sugar syrup. Honey heated to improve the flow through industrial equipment is degraded in 'soul' quality. All is called organic because the bees are 'wild'.

True, bees that suck from heavily sprayed crops don't make it back to the hive, so most honey is pretty clean. The best quality honey comes from remote virgin forest, so inaccessible sometimes that the hives are delivered and collected on pallets by helicopter. But you still have to question the processing after harvest.

Go for set honey, and be reassured by streaks of whiter crystals visible inside the glass jar. These indicate traditional, cool handling. Local beekeepers are an honest breed, and often sell good produce through local shops, labelled with their address.

In any case, use honey very sparingly, chiefly as a spread on bread.

JAM Technically this must have 60 per cent sugar to ensure safe preservation, so use very little (as a spread perhaps). Conserves with less or no sugar have to be refrigerated once opened, but are almost all fruit. These are readily available from health shops and well worth the extra cost.

JUICE Generally you are better off eating the fresh raw fruit (or vegetable), or juicing it yourself at home. This is a good use of fallen or marked fruit, for example. You will pay a lot to buy a manufactured product of that quality, which is next favourite. The juice is intensely flavoursome – a bomb in your mouth – and you won't want to drink large quantities, so it's still good value. Juices made from boiled-down juice concentrate, and sold by the ton in cardboard bricks, are far and away less good value – as you can tell from the weaker flavour. You can drink it by the glassful with scarcely any impact.

Make or buy a little fresh raw juice to start your meal, by all means. Leave the other stuff alone. The exception would be the organic cartoned juices, which when diluted are a good substitute for cordial and squash.

KIDNEY This is the organ by which the animal excretes anything undesirable, so beware of eating any produced intensively. In fact, it's best avoided if you have gut problems.

KIPPER Smoked herring is a great delicacy, the ideal protein breakfast. Don't buy them coloured, or small – we must all discourage the fishing of immature stock. Best grilled quickly – 2 minutes on the back, 3 on the front – and eaten alone – no bread. You can eat the bread afterwards, if you are still hungry – but you probably won't be.

KIWI FRUIT I don't think this has much more than cosmetic value. It comes from half way around the world, tastes a bit limp and is probably sprayed heavily.

LARD The only good use for this saturated animal fat is to fry meat or pancakes without their sticking to the pan. That accounts for about an ounce a year. Otherwise avoid it.

LEEK A great indigenous, substantial vegetable of the onion family that is available fresh throughout a long winter season. Easy to grow organically in your garden, and well worth it. The tenderest hearts may be eaten raw but they're usually better steamed a little, whole, as part of your vegetable course.

LENTIL A very rich protein source containing starch, so the soaked boiled seeds (whole or split) are indigestible. Better to buy them whole and sprout them.

You soak them overnight, then rinse and drain them twice or three times daily, and keep them in jars on a warm windowsill. After two to three days a shoot grows the length of the lentil, inside its skin. Once it's about to break out, you can eat the lentils raw or wok them. The longer the shoot, the stringier it becomes.

LIVER This is the main chemical factory of the body, and very rich food – but in intensively reared livestock, concentrates toxic residues too. Only buy from organic animals. In the long run, learn to live without it.

MARGARINE The original versions based on animal or coconut fat can be discarded, along with lard. They have little relevance or value in the modern world.

Many vegetable margarines include a little dairy fat to aid emulsification, so if you are dairy-sensitive read labels with care.

The rape and sunflower oils used are partially hydrogenated, and in the process make 'trans' (opposite side) bonds that are unnatural and unhealthy. The natural 'cis' (same side) bonds are preserved in natural oils, of which sunflower, wheatgerm and olive oil are the best. Make a thick spreadable mayonnaise from one of these for the safest, most tasty, margarine substitute.

MARMALADE Made with whole oranges, it includes the fungicides on the peel, intended to prevent rot in transit – not to be eaten. Only ever accept organic marmalade, because these fungicides sometimes cause gut pain – even in people without a chronic problem. If you make your own, buy organic Seville oranges.

MARMITE™ see spread

MARROW, VEGETABLE The least worthwhile of the large vegetable fruits in this family, in my opinion. Even the organic ones taste of very little. They make a good wine, I am told, and can be stuffed with something more flavoursome as a vegetable course or vegetarian main dish. You're better off with pumpkin.

MAYONNAISE A thick, tasty, spreadable sauce can be made as follows as a wholesome substitute for butter and manufactured margarine:

- Beat some salt, pepper and 1 teaspoon of pure mustard powder (ideally mustard seeds in a spice mill) with the yolk of 1 free-range egg and 1 teaspoonful of organic cider vinegar, both at room temperature.

- Very gradually, add cool organic oil – olive and/ or sunflower. At first do so drop by drop, blending continuously (but not too fast), letting each drop emulsify before adding the next.
- Once the emulsion has gelled, add another teaspoonful of vinegar, and then the remaining oil a little faster, until it has thickened – about 150ml (5 fl oz).
- Use more or less vinegar to obtain the thickness you want.

MEAT, FRESH

I live in a small market town blessed with excellent butchers, whom I would happily patronise more if I were surer of their livestock sources. For the present, none of us are. We know far too little about the transmissibility and extent of BSE, and should be wary of official reassurances about it for a good while yet.

Well cut pork and lamb are, nevertheless, good choices and Scottish beef is usually free-range and virtually organic. No organic producers have yet suffered BSE, so far as I know, so mail order organic specialists (with the right certificates) should be trustworthy.

Wild game is a better bet, when available.

MELON

A ripe honeydew melon is delicious, and makes a good first course. Watermelon is basically water and less flavoursome. Both are overpriced for their limited nutritive value, because they are not easy to grow. Organic versions are hard to come by.

MILK

Cows' milk is one route by which the animal dumps toxins it has been forced to eat, most of which are fat-soluble; so skimmed milk (no fat) is safer. This is no defence if you are genuinely cow-sensitive, of course, since all the allergenic protein is the watery part.

Soya milk bears no resemblance to any dairy item, except colour and fluidity. It contains more aluminium than most plants and until we know more about the effects of long-term exposure I advise against that. Some gut problems can be traced to aluminium exposure, certainly.

The best cow substitute is the goat, whose milk resembles human milk much more closely anyway.

However, milk is not a particularly appropriate food after about two years of age. Humans are unique in consuming it outside infancy, let alone from another animal. Drink it if you like it, but don't feel obliged.

You can get readily available calcium from fresh nuts and vegetables instead.

'MINCE'
This is what's left after the butcher has taken all the decent cuts. After what I said about meat, you can draw your own conclusion. If this is all you can afford, save your money.

MINCEMEAT (SWEET)
This rich mixture of suet, sugar, vine fruits and spices bears practically no resemblance to the meat preserve of former centuries. Mince tarts are tasty but very wicked. You've no idea what pollutants are dissolved in the suet. If you've gut problems, give this a miss.

MINT
This is a useful cooking herb for people with gut problems, combining fragrance with soothing digestive properties. Hence the fashion for after-dinner mints, which you should avoid. Grow a mint variety at home in a pot and make liberal use of it.

MOUSSE
This confection of milk, gelatine and sugar combines three dangerous items in one mouthful. You are best advised to avoid this and all other dainty desserts.

MUESLI
The original idea was to make coarsely rolled raw oats digestible by eating them with grated fresh fruit and raw milk. None of the modern offerings get anywhere near this, and most add sugar you do not need. Make up your own, using nuts, seed and dried fruit to taste along with rolled organic oats, but eat a piece of fresh fruit before or along with it.

Moisten it sparingly with milk, to retain a good crumb structure on the spoon. You can follow it with more bread or toast, but nothing else.

MUSHROOM
These fungi (related to yeasts) offer texture and a delicious but subtle flavour, but not much nourishment. Always choose organic, though – this crop is intensively sprayed otherwise.

People with a *Candida* problem can usually eat mushrooms safely (Chapter Six). They offer an extra flavour variety if your range of staple foods is limited. To be eaten as vegetables or included in casseroles and sauces – cooked well, by all means, if you have yeast problems.

MUSSELS
See shellfish

MUSTARD
This hot, leggy salad leaf may be eaten with cress (to dilute its impact) as a first course, but the seeds are better known as the basis of Europe's favourite relish (outside Italy). It goes well with ham and smoked fish and is a valuable ingredient in scrambled egg, mayonnaise and vinaigrette. You can use whole mustard seed in a spice grinder, as a condiment alongside (or instead of) pepper and salt.

NUT

(See also peanut.) All seeds are comprehensive, concentrated rations to get a new plant started in life, and nuts are simply the large seeds of trees. All are valuable live foods to try. Only buy whole nut kernels: broken pieces may be cheaper but they go stale and mouldy very easily.

Use them as the basis of a main vegetarian dish, or nibble them as your live first course.

Peanuts are more peas than nuts.

OAT, PORRIDGE

This staple fare of northern Europe is related to wheat, and grown in poorer soils that will not yield wheat well. The grains are softer and roll out well, but the process of separating the unpalatable husk is quite complex, so the millers earn their keep well. How Scottish crofters ever managed I don't know.

This is the best breakfast cereal, and readily available organically grown. You are probably better to look for it in health shops. Cook it with water and perhaps a little salt: add milk and copped fruit as you serve it. You can mix extra raw bran into porridge as you make it, if you feel the need.

OIL

Natural oil from seeds, fruits and fish are valuable foods, contain fatty acids essential for human health. They mainly come in two chemically distinct varieties – omega-3 (e.g. linoleic acid) from oily fish, dark green leaves and linseed; and omega-6 (e.g. linolenic acid) from other seeds. (The omega business is just a chemical notation for locating the position of the unsaturated bonds in the molecule – the number of bonds in from the end of the string.)

So always have in some good, traditional vegetable oil – wheatgerm, sunflower, peanut – even if you use it only sparingly in dressings for salad and in cooking. Don't deep-fry with it – you degrade the oil into something more irritant and dangerous. In fact, don't deep-fry.

I am wary of safflower and rape oil because they are not traditional foods, however much omega-6 fatty acid they contain. Olive oil, on the other hand, is especially to my taste and I use it freely on that account, despite its lower essential fatty acid content.

Avoid oils that do not advertise their vegetable of origin – they probably come from the coconut palm, and don't provide anything essential.

Fish body oil is now available as an omega-3 food supplement, quite distinct from fish liver oil. Most people get sufficient from the whole oily fish – mackerel, herring etc – whether fresh or smoked.

OLIVE

(See also Oil.) Doubtless olives get sprayed just like most other things, but they are still the most innocent of cocktail nibbles and are welcome in most salads. Like wine, they vary subtly in flavour according to their origin, which adds interest. They are also quite nourishing, and I have yet to hear of anybody being allergic to them. No, don't bother to write . . .

ONION

This is possibly the most useful vegetable of all, and second only to greens in value. Organic onions are easy to obtain and well worth the premium. If you have problems digesting them, beware also of leeks, chives and garlic – all of the same family. You may find that boiled or braised onions go down better than fried or baked. Eat with your vegetable course.

ORANGE

The taste of fruit delivered in northern Europe bears very little resemblance to those eaten in their countries of origin, so quite a lot is lost in transit. They are often gassed in their containers, as well as sprayed, so they are seldom chemical-free. Citrus fruit is sometimes blamed for stomach acidity, but I am sure it's really the pollutant chemicals.

Northerners may have trouble coping with the amount of juice and fruit available without some sensitivity problems – we get on better with grapes, apples and pears that are native here.

PARSLEY

This is the richest leaf vegetable known, as well as one of the strongest-flavoured. So it is used as a herbal garnish, which may be as well since (like celery, its relative) it contains psoralens – chemicals considered carcinogenic. I suspect that the nourishment in parsley is more than a match for that, so continue to use leaves from a couple of plants in pots.

PARSNIP

Related to parsley but used only for its roots, since its leaves are too strongly flavoured and perhaps mildly poisonous – they contain psoralens, which I presume are also in the roots. If you have a passion for parsnips, try to contain it to a few meals around Christmas.

PASTA

The Italian way to prepare wheat, but far harder to separate from the rich sauces with which it is often served, so not easy to digest well. If you have gut problems, make sure to eat only wholemeal, organic pasta, right at the end of the meal – otherwise give it a miss.

PASTE

This catch-all covers tomato, meat, fish, soya- and yeast-based offerings. In general, you do not know what you are getting. Leave the meat ones alone, and avoid any that are packed in metal tubes. Yeast is probably the least adulterated, since there is so much available cheaply from the brewing industry. Tomato paste is the most desirable, and may just be worth risking the metal tube.

PASTRY If you value your digestion, don't risk it.

PEANUT More pea than nut. Walnuts, brazils and hazels (filberts) are more expensive but more digestible and better food.

PEAR Nobody ever seems to become allergic to pears. They are less digestible than apples until they are very ripe and soft, when they make a good raw first course.

PEAS The sugar in this popular summer vegetable is not a problem when they are young, but becomes more so as they age and go starchy. That combined with protein makes for difficult digestion. Sprout dried peas (see lentil) before use, to overcome that problem.

PEPPER (CONDIMENT) If you enjoy seasoned food, obtain a spice grinder and a supply of peppercorns and do the job properly. You will be more sparing, which is good.

PEPPER (FRUIT) An excellent fruit for savoury salads and vegetable casseroles, related to the tomato and potato. The different colours indicate their high antioxidant content, and change as they ripen. A good raw item to start any meal with.

PESTO Based on parmesan cheese and basil, this traditional accompaniment to pasta is also a pleasant relish on salads and green vegetables.

PICKLE Preserving in vinegar produces a durable, sour result which you are probably best to avoid. As a method of food conservation it is long superseded, but gherkins, onions and walnuts improve for pickling, according to some.

PIGEONS See game.

PISTACHIO The best nibbling nut. The time it takes to shell them puts a brake on your consumption.

PORRIDGE See oats.

POTATO This now rivals wheat as our staple source of energy, but provides far less fibre unless you eat the skins. The outer 5mm (¼″) is both the most nourishing part and the most polluted by sprays, so organic potatoes are well worth their premium. Much more digestible than cereal but still best eaten at the very end of the meal, the starch course.

Don't ever eat potatoes with green patches under the skin. They have been exposed to the sun and produced a bitter poison (solanine) which stops rats eating them, but it will also provoke acute gut trouble.

Chips absorb lots of fat that has been heated sufficiently to alter its chemical structure. The result is less
valuable nutritionally and a potential irritant to the gut.
Bake your potatoes dry in the oven instead. Even a pat
of butter on top is less harmful than the quality and
quantity of fat in chips.

PRUNE
Both dried and fresh plums help invigorate a flabby
bowel muscle, so include them in your first course
(second after fresh juice) at breakfast if you are
inclined to get constipated.

PUDDING
The savoury varieties – black, from blood, and white,
from offal – are best avoided for the moment. Suet
pudding is intended to sustain regular hard physical
labour, and is redundant now – quite apart from the
pollution potential of suet (the special fat round the
kidney). Christmas pudding (plum duff) and summer
pudding are delicious, but awkward combinations to
digest – even as the last course of the meal – and quite
fattening. Summer pudding is marginally safer than
the rest.

PUMPKIN
American cousin of the vegetable marrow and vastly
superior in flavour, value and cooking possibility.
Makes excellent soup and custard substitute (commonly in pies, see Pastry). The seeds are good nibbles.
Since pumpkins are usually grown on a smallholding
scale with lots of compost, the seeds have a better
mineral content – notably potassium, iron and zinc –
than most other field crops. As their colour indicates,
they are loaded with antioxidant vitamin A.

RABBIT
Better than intensive poultry but wild is best. See
Game.

RAISINS
The best way to obtain the mineral value of grapes
without the spray risk – so long as you buy them
organic, of course.

RHUBARB
Looks like the dessert version of celery, but a different
plant family. Of very little food value and liable to
contain oxalic acid – a no-no if you suffer kidney
stones. But the juice is quite good for getting your
bowel to move.

RICE
Distant relative of wheat, barley, oats and maize, but
not so nourishing as the first three even when eaten
whole – which it usually is not. Basmati rice is the
most nourishing. The habit of eating it with Indian or
Chinese dishes is a Western invention – the Chinese
only eat rice last, if still hungry, just as I recommend.
In general, bad value for people with gut problems.

ROE
Being fish eggs (hard) or sperm(soft) this is a valuable
protein, particularly if you are pregnant or trying to

conceive. Cook very gently – no frying! – to conserve the value of your purchase.

SALMON

See fish, gravadlax. There is much more salmon available now because considerable stocks are farmed in sea enclosures. This can be well or badly done, and we have no means yet of knowing which you are buying. Go by the firmness and flavour of the meat, and stick with brands that particularly impress you. Better still, visit a few salmon farms whilst on holiday and see what you think of them. Then be loyal to the most impressive. Wild is always likely to be best of all.

Support the Scots and Irish industries, who have always in the past done an excellent job. 'Irish/ Scottish Smoked Salmon' may have been farmed or caught elsewhere – you want 'Smoked Irish/Scottish Salmon'.

SALT (CONDIMENT)

Don't be afraid to use up to a teaspoonful of salt in various forms daily. It's essential for health, and you can easily take too little trying to keep your blood pressure down. Use sea-salt for authenticity and iodine.

SAUSAGE

A more familiar form of white pudding, it usually contains rusk (biscuit) as well as minced meat offals. This is inherently indigestible, apart from questions about the nutritional value and safety of the undeclared ingredients. Give them up. If you can't, there are some more expensive organic varieties available with no rusk, which you could buy occasionally to appease the craving.

SHELLFISH

Once the staple protein food of the London poor, their price has gone up but they remain good value.

Including them in salads, or on brown bread, is not a good idea. It's far better to base your main protein course on them, or use a few to garnish it. Shelling them as you eat slows you down, which is always good.

SOYA

See also Bean. The soya bean is grown on a huge scale and marketed heavily for many purposes – industrial food processing, meat substitutes (TVP), milk substitutes, desserts and tofu. Large quantities are used as primary sources of chemicals and pharmaceuticals, particularly in hormone manufacture.

A few people still buy the whole beans and just cook them. That's the sensible way to prepare them in Europe – get them organic and GM-free. Tofu and bean curd belong to an oriental culture you can emulate if you wish, but they're not superior to whole beans.

Nor is soya better than lentils and other beans. The particularly high protein content (like lentils) makes them even more indigestible than other beans, unless you sprout them. See also 'Milk'.

SPICES These hot and highly flavoured seeds were traditionally used, in the days before refrigeration, to disguise meat that is beginning to rot. Now they are used to flavour mass-produced meats that have none of their own!

They can easily upset your gut so use them sparingly if you have problems. It's another incentive to buy decent free-range, organic meat in the first place.

SPINACH A plentiful source of green leaves, faster-growing and therefore less valuable than the cabbage family but more valuable than lettuce.

SPREAD, SAVOURY See also paste. Protein spreads on bread are dangerous digestive ground – you must have gathered that by now – so avoid them all. Use vegetable spread in mayonnaise, or similar, instead.

You could use the protein spreads to flavour hot savoury drinks or soup, however. In general, the safest of these are based on yeast, which is an abundant waste product of the brewing trade. For the present, products that look very similar but are derived from slaughter house waste are far less desirable.

SQUASH See Cordial/Pumpkin

SUET See also pudding. This is special fat from around the kidneys, prized in the past but now just as dubious value as lard.

SUGAR You should not be buying a bag of sugar more than once in a blue moon. Beware also of the sugar included in manufactured items – baked beans, for example, and soup. Look also on the ingredient label for sucrose, glucose, dried or hydrogenated glucose syrup, hydrogenated high maltose glucose syrup, dextrose, fructose, invert sugar, isomalt, lactose, maltose and xylitol – avoid them all. They can all work havoc among the germ colonies in your caecum.

SULTANAS See Raisins

SWEETCORN See Corn

SWEETS See Confectionery/Dessert

TOMATO I feel sorry for people who cannot cope with this great salad fruit standby. Grow them yourself or buy organic, before deciding you are 'allergic' to them. They are related to peppers and aubergines, so you may get away with those instead. They are loaded with antioxidant carotenoids – relatives of vitamin A.

Good in your raw first course, or as a vegetable to follow. Fairly safe in a mixed grill or a home-made sauce in your main course, but it's wisest to eat grilled tomatoes (and mushrooms) before tackling the meaty items.

TROUT
Alas, most trout is intensively farmed and medicated – sometimes even coloured: not good news for your gut problem. You are better off with salmon, or any fresh sea fish.

TURKEY
An import from America, very inbred and utterly reliant on human help to survive – so a rather sorry species. The meat is, however, usually firmer and tastier than chicken, which may mean turkey is less intensively farmed. I certainly hope so. You're still better off with game, eaten more occasionally.

VEGETABLE BOUILLON, SWISS
This is available organically produced, or low-salt, to suit your preference. It is an ideal basis for soup or a hot savoury drink. I use it all the time.

VEGETABLE MARGARINE
See Margarine

VENISON
It's actually quite ecological to eat deer-meat. Wild deer have no natural enemies and need to be culled occasionally, to control numbers. The trade in carcasses is carefully regulated, ending with the High Street game-dealer. Some venison is now farmed, unfortunately, which creates the temptation and opportunity to tamper with it. This is more likely to end up on the slab of an ordinary butcher or supermarket.

VINEGAR
Wine and cider vinegar are both available organically, and are strong enough to make good mayonnaise or vinaigrette. The latter may be sufficient to help reinforce deficient stomach acid, if consumed with your protein course.

You can flavour a hot drink with it. In combination with good honey, a very old folk medicine whose principle virtue is its comprehensive mineral content, though in very tiny amounts.

WINE
Apart from its pleasing flavour and alcohol content, wine safely preserves the rich mineral and antioxidant content of grapes, so is (in moderation) a legitimate food. But it must be properly made, not chemical plonk. Buy only good wine and drink less of it.

YOGHURT
The way goats' milk ferments naturally, yoghurt was for centuries a convenient way to conserve it in the countries around the Mediterranean. It can be contrived in cows' milk, but does not come naturally.

It's not the dairy solid in yoghurt that is healthy, but the live germs that soured it. Therefore pasteurised yoghurt is of no health value – don't buy it.

'Natural' refers to the flavour, not the germ content. You need live or unpasteurised yoghurt if you want to get your caecum working well. To test it, put a teaspoon in some warm milk and check that it curdles and goes sour in a few hours. If not, don't buy it again.

The good ones usually announce the live bug count (in millions) on the label.

Chapter Ten: Special Diets

Once you have got thoroughly used to the principles outlined so far, you will seldom, if ever, have to resort to anything more specialised. However, there are a few situations which may call for additional help, which are these.

THE CLEANSING DIET

Most people nowadays eat lots of the kinds of food that contain chemicals your body will have difficulty getting rid of. These include pesticides and other agricultural chemicals in fresh items like vegetables and fruit, meat and cheese, as well as chemical additives in manufactured, processed and refined products such as confectionery, biscuits, bread, sugar, packet soups and desserts (Chapter Five). For the average person in Britain today the E-coded chemicals and artificial flavourings alone add up to the equivalent of 18 tablets of soluble aspirin every day!

We know that many food chemicals are poisonous in any quantity and we can assume that even small amounts of each chemical, acting along with the 3000 or so other chemicals we consume daily, are together irritant enough to nag at our guts and make them more prone to disease. To cap all this, the acidic material, left over after digestion of protein in the liver, stays in the blood for some time before you can get rid of it. If you eat protein faster than you can get rid of these waste acids they build up in the blood, creating traffic congestion which delays and interferes with all your body's self-cleansing activities. If you ever get 'muscular rheumatism' – a fleeting pain that goes away if you move or massage the muscle – you are probably building up protein residues in this way. (Cramp is different, and more likely a mineral imbalance.)

Dr Max Bircher-Benner worked all this out and devised a successful means of dealing with many diseases through diet and hydrotherapy. A trial of his method was conducted at the Royal Free Hospital in 1936 involving the twelve most chronic, bed-ridden rheumatoid arthritis cases under Dr Dorothy Hare's care. Seven of them carried their own suitcases home within weeks. Only two were beyond help.

More recently, Professor Arnold Ehret devised a 'mucusless' diet for reducing the level of waste acid (mucus) in the body, and it is this version of Bircher-Benner's treatment that I recommend to people today for independent home use.

When victims of accumulative diseases make the effort to cut down on their mucus build-up and chemical pollution by improving their diets, they often benefit far more than from medicines they may be offered. Incidentally, they often discover a much higher level of energy and efficiency that they hadn't realised they'd lost.

Preparing for Fitness

All this is particularly important if you want to get fit again to enjoy an active sport. A lot of people now realise how important it is to get reasonably fit before they start to play a sport vigorously, but far fewer would-be sports-people understand that they should clean up their bodies carefully first, even before they try to get fit.

Increased activity in a chemically dirty body puts it under much greater stress, and may threaten its health. The only safe thing to do is get your body clean first, before you set about getting fit.

The diet that follows is designed to achieve this for you, whether for sport or for overcoming accumulative disease including IBS. Read through the whole scheme before you attempt it. If you have doubts relating to your particular condition, check with your doctor before beginning. You can phone WellDesk (see Useful Addresses) if you need further help after that.

The Diet

1. Prepare by cutting out:
   - sugar in any form (beware the large amounts hidden in processed foods – READ THE LABELS and see below for more details)

- white or refined flour in any form – only organic wholemeal is a real improvement
- coffee and strong Indian tea; cocoa, cola and chocolate are also very unhelpful in any quantity.

2. If you really mean business, begin with a two-day fast on home-made barley water (see p. 124) or fresh diluted fruit juice (mineral or filtered tap-water). Do not be put off if so little food makes you feel ill, but take time off work if necessary. You have 'flu', which arises just as often from a bodily 'spring clean' as from a virus infection – the two are indistinguishable. An illness like this does not usually take more than a week, and shows how urgently you need cleansing. But it takes nerve: support from a doctor or WellDesk (see Useful Addresses) is very valuable.

3. After two days start eating one or two pieces of fresh fruit at mealtimes. Apples and bananas are very suitable. You can add or substitute any raw vegetable for variety. Do this for several days more.

4. When you feel well and hungry, commence two meals a day – a late breakfast or lunch, and an evening meal. Drink juice or barley water between meals as desired, but not during, or for an hour, after-eating. *There is no need to go hungry.*

5. Breakfast: Start if you wish with a cup of juniper berry tea prepared overnight, or freshly brewed broom or parsley piert. All these herbs promote cleansing of your blood, through the kidneys. Proceed to a generous fresh fruit course, as many pieces as you wish in any variety. Pause for a few minutes, and if you are still genuinely hungry, eat dry organic wholemeal toast, or mixed nuts and raisins, until you are satisfied.

6. Main meal: start with a generous fresh coleslaw including cabbage, onion and carrot. Obtain organically grown vegetables if at all possible, to avoid eating more of the chemicals you are trying to get rid off. Pause, then have one sort of baked vegetable of your choice: potatoes, a root variety, beans (not from a tin), broccoli or cauliflower. Cook them gently and slowly in a closed dish, in their own juice.

7. After three weeks you should be ready for a more normal diet (Chapter Eight), avoiding routinely the items you now realise are unwholesome. You can then afford to take part in occasional celebrations and restaurant outings without expecting mishap.

8. Call the WellDesk helpline (see Useful Addresses) for personal guidance by professional health advisers, supervised by a doctor. You should, of course, always ask your own doctor for assistance.

9. If you still have gut problems after this, or they return with a more normal diet, you should check for specific food sensitivities. (see p. 158)

10. An occasional exposure to a pesticide or other chemical may upset you exceptionally, out of the blue, even months after you have got rid of your IBS. You can safely use garlic oil to flush it out – 2 mg with plenty of water before meals, twice daily for two days. Call WellDesk (see Useful Addresses) for details.

WEIGHT CONTROL

It is easy to understand why so many people get fat. A rich diet of counterfeit food deranges your appetite; you crave exactly the wrong things because they have you hooked. You exercise little because you have no time to walk or cycle everywhere, or live too far from work and the best shops. Yet constant stress makes you long for relief sometimes and nice food is an inexpensive, portable and socially acceptable substitute for anything better. You join a large minority of Westerners of all ages, five to 15 kilograms overweight with lumps of fat under your shoulderblades and around your waist. Your complexion is waxier than you would like, marred further perhaps by cheesy blackheads or septic spots.

So you start on a reducing diet. There are any number to choose from, all based on the idea of reducing your consumption of fuel – calories – to less than you need each day. The initial weight loss is impressive but unreal. Burning off old fat comes next, and is not so easy. Any alternative diet of the same kind has exactly the same effect. Indeed, you may tend to gain a little weight overall after finishing each attempt.

Hard work may help, if you are short of exercise and not over-tired physically already. But no one ever lost weight by exercise alone. Exercise turns some of your fat into muscle, which shapes and hardens you up, but that spare tyre will only yield fully to a proper diet combined with exercise.

The key to this lies not in the calorie theory at all, but in combining foods properly within your meals. There are certain definite 'do's' and 'don'ts' but the key principle to understand is how your body puts on fat in the first place.

When you eat food that makes sugar in your blood this provokes a hormone called insulin which stores the sugar in muscle and other tissues that can use it. If the surge of blood sugar is smooth and gradual (as with wholemeal cereals and most fruits) the insulin matches it exactly and no surplus remains. If, however, the sugar surge is torrential, the insulin response is out of proportion, and an extra amount remains in the blood after all the sugar is stored. This amount is used up by storing any fat that is in your blood, whether from the same meal or an earlier one, as fat in your body tissue. That is your spare tyre, the thickening of your skin around the middle and under your shoulder-blades.

So the secrets of losing surplus weight are two-fold. Do not eat foods which cause a strong, sudden surge of sugar into your blood; and never eat starchy food in the same meal as vegetable oils or fatty food.

You can eat fats and oils with protein, when no harm is done. You can eat starchy food with anything but protein or fat. It is the combination that does the damage. It really is, in principle, as simple as that.

What to do

1. Weight charts cannot cater for individual build or muscle mass, so read them with caution. Skin-fold thickness cal-lipers are a more reliable measure of fat, but hard to use accurately without help. Modern scales that also measure body impedance are probably the easiest to use: you get a figure for the percentage of your body which is fat. If your

body fat proportion is over 22 per cent, or your Body Mass Index (calculated from your height and weight, using tables) is higher than 35 and you are not in training as a weight-lifter, you are probably carrying excess fat.

2. Do not try to diet during pregnancy. You will do better well covered, and start feeding it to your baby after about four months' lactation; so breast-feeding for at least six months gets rid of it.

3. The starchy foods always to be wary of are sugar in any form, refined (white or granary) bread, flour and cereals, potatoes and bananas. Wholemeal bread (not malt loaf, croissants or pastries), oats, shredded wheat and whole rye crackers are fine. Beans are good starches for cooking. Strong coffee increases the blood sugar, so beware of that.

4. Breakfast: wholemeal toast with sugar-free jam (no fatty spread), plain porridge, shredded wheat with skimmed milk or any combination of these is ideal. You can occasionally have boiled or poached eggs or fish (no bread with either) or a slap-up mixed grill (protein and fat) but exclude bread, toast, chips, fried bread, baked beans and hash browns.

5. Start every main meal with a generous raw salad or cole-slaw, using olive, wheatgerm or sunflower oil with cider vinegar or lemon juice as a dressing. Chew it well and slowly, and pause for a few minutes before eating your next course. If you don't feel hungry any more, don't proceed. Eggs, meat, fish or vegetables with salad (no bread, carrots, turnips, parsnips or potatoes) are appropriate main courses. Cheese or yoghurt is permissible as dessert – no crackers.

6. Exercise gently for ten minutes three times a week at first to get reasonably fit, then work it up to 30 minutes. Do something you enjoy, vary it if you get bored, and try to make it useful. Perhaps you could cycle to work. This will keep you burning fat and stop you hibernating (see Slow Metabolism, p. 102).

7. If faithful adherence to this does not result in weight loss within a fortnight, you should ask your doctor whether you need a thyroid check. Depending on his response you may need to contact WellDesk (see Useful Addresses) for help about possible hibernation.

TESTING, TESTING: EXCLUSION DIETS

Food allergy or intolerance is not the cause of every problem, but it proves to be an important contributor to illness in quite a few people, including up to one in ten children. However, standard medical allergy tests do not work on foods as a rule, so you need a reliable trick for spotting the trouble yourself.

The difficulties with food allergy tests trace back to how stress reacts on people. At first your body protests vigorously, trying to reject the stress. In a few weeks however, everything seems to return to normal – but there is one more burden on your health-keeping budget. If you are just about coping but grumbling, you are compensating from reserves: that will eventually run you down. So you look for stresses you can change, and food is clearly high on that list. Relieve a food stress and you increase your ability to cope with other stresses over which you have less control: result, a better life.

What to do
1. To discover whether foods or chemicals are responsible for chronic symptoms you have, you need to eat none of the suspect food for just four days, then reintroduce it. Monday morning until Friday afternoon is convenient, reintroducing the test food at teatime on Friday. Any reaction will be over in time to test something else next week.
2. To be sure of a clear result you must eat nothing in those four days that could deputise for the food you are testing. This means in practice that you must exclude all members of the same biological family at the same time. Here are the families that most commonly prove to be troublesome:

- THE COW: beef, suet, beef stock cubes, Oxo™, Bovril™, milk chocolate; items including dried skimmed milk, casein, whey powder, milk solids, cow's milk, butter, cream, yoghurt, cheese.
- CEREALS: wheat, wheat flour of all kinds, wheat bran, semolina; packaged items including wheat, gluten, or flour. Strictly speaking, barley, oats, rye, maize, millet, rice, sweetcorn and sugar all belong here too, but strict exclusion of all wheat and sugar usually works in practice;

you can replace them with potatoes, or a little of the other cereals you do not usually eat.

- GLUTEN: wheat (including that advertised as 'gluten free', which may still contain up to 2 per cent of gluten), barley, oats, rye.
- POTATO: potato, tomato, aubergine, pepper (cayenne, chillies, paprika, pimento), ground cherry, physalis, tobacco.
- HEN: chicken, hen's egg, chicken stock cubes.
- DRINKS: coffee, tea (Indian, China and Sri Lankan), chocolate, cocoa, cola.
- SALICYLATES: aspirin, several classes of food additives (colourings, benzoates, hydroxybenzoates, gallates, trihydroxybenzoates); almonds, apple, apricot, blackberry, blackcurrant, cherry, cider vinegar, cucumber, currant, gooseberry, grape, lemon, marrow, peach, pepper, plum, prune, orange, raisin, raspberry, rosehip, strawberry, sultana, tangerine, tomato, wine vinegar.
- CITRUS: grapefruit, lemon, lime, mandarin, orange, tangerine.

3. You may improve during the exclusion but expect no change. However, after reintroduction of an item that has been troubling you, an obvious reaction may occur in 20 minutes–12 hours. Record it exactly in detail, while it is vivid. Record the negative findings just as carefully, of course.
4. Carry on excluding foods from families you reacted to, but go back to eating those that proved safe.

If you seem, after many weeks of testing, to be allergic to lots of food families, your immune system needs a general overhaul. Consult a professional health practitioner or doctor.

The following list of a wide range of foods is classified into biological families, and you may be able to make up a few extra tests by reference to it. More usefully, you will be able to find which foods you can safely substitute for staples you have decided to exclude long-term. So long as your choice is from a separate family, there should be no deputisation or cross-sensitivity.

Food families
Plants

Aizoaceae: New Zealand spinach
Anacardiaceae: cashew, pistachio, mango
Betulaceae: hazelnut, filbert
Caricaceae: pawpaw
Chenopodiaceae: beetroot, spinach, sugar beet, Swiss chard
Compositae: artichoke (globe and Jerusalem), chamomile, chicory, dandelion, endive, lettuce, safflower, salsify, scorzonera, sunflower, tarragon
Convolvulaceae: sweet potato
Cruciferae: Brussels sprout, broccoli, cabbage, cauliflower, Chinese cabbage, horseradish, kale, kohl rabi, landcress, mustard, radish, rape, swede, turnip, watercress
Cucurbitaceae: cantaloop, cucumber, courgette, marrow, melon, pumpkin, squash, water melon
Cycadaceae: sago
Dioscoreaceae: yam
Ebenaceae: persimmon
Ericaceae: bilberry, blueberry, cranberry, damson, huckleberry, sloe
Euphorbiaceae: cassava, tapioca
Fugaceae: sweet chestnut
Fungi: mushroom, yeast, Marmite™
Gramineae: bamboo shoot, barley, sweetcorn, maize, millet, oat, rice, rye, sugar cane, wheat
Juglandaceae: walnut, hicory nut, butter nut
Labiatae: balm, basil, hoarhound, mint, marjoram, oregano, peppermint, spearmint, rosemary, sage, savory, thyme
Laurus: herb teas
Leguminosae: dry beans, green beans, lentils, liquorice, pea, peanut
Liliaceae: asparagus, olive, garlic, leek, onion, shallot
Malvaceae: okra
Marantaceae: arrowroot
Moraceae: mulberry, fig, bread fruit
Murtaceae: guava
Musaceae: banana, plantain
Oleaceae: olive, olive oil

Onagraceae: water chestnut
Palmae: coconut, date
Passifloraceae: passion fruit
Polygonaceae: buckwheat, rhubarb
Portulacaceae: Miner's lettuce
Rosaceae: apple, apricot, blackberry, cherry, loganberry, nectarine, peach, pear, plum, prune, raspberry, rosehip, strawberry
Rubiaceae: coffee
Rutaceae: grapefruit, lemon, lime, mandarin, orange, tangerine
Saxifragaceae: gooseberry, black and red currant
Solanaceae: aubergine, cayenne, chilli, ground cherry, paprika, (sweet) pepper, pimento, potato, physalis, tobacco, tomato
Theaceae: Indian or China tea
Torreya: nutmeg, mace, Brazil nut
Umbelliferae: angelica, anice, caraway, carrot, celeriac, celery, coriander, dill, fennel, parsley, parsnip, samphire
Valerianaceae: lamb's lettuce
Vitaceae: grapes, vine, peppercorn.

Animals

Anatidae: duck, duck eggs, goose, goose eggs
Bovidae: beef, suet, beef stock cube, Oxo™, Bovril™, milk chocolate, cow's milk, butter, cream, yoghurt, cheese, dairy ice-cream; any item containing dried skimmed milk, casein, whey powder, milk solids
Caprinae: goat meat, kid, milk, cheese, yoghurt; sheep's milk, cheese, lamb, mutton
Cervidae: venison
Columbidae: pigeon, dove
Crustaceanae: crab, crayfish, lobster, prawn, shrimp
Leporidae: hare, rabbit
Meleagrinae: turkey
Molluscae: abalone, clam, mussel, oyster, scallop, snail, squid
Phasianidae: partridge, pheasant, chicken, chicken stock cube, hen's egg
Ranidae: edible frog
Scolopacidae: snipe, woodcock
Suidae: pork, ham, bacon, pig's liver, pork sausage
Tetraonidae: grouse, ptarmigan, capercaillie

Turnicidae: quail*, quail's eggs (* Quail in the wild are protected by law. Hunting them or robbing their nests is an offence.)

Fishes

Asipenseridae: sturgeon, caviar
Anguilliformes: eel
Clupeidae: herring, anchovy
Cyprinidae: carp
Gadiformes: cod, haddock
Merluccuidae: hake
Mugiladae: mullet
Percoidei: bass, perch, sea bream
Pleuronectidae: plaice, halibut, flounder
Rajidae: skate
Salmoniformes: trout, salmon
Scombridae: tuna, mackerel
Soleidae: sole

CUTTING DOWN ON SUGAR

Coronaries and arteriosclerosis, stomach ulcers, varicose veins and constipation are all 'saccharine diseases', as well as diabetes and dental disease. These are all now a serious risk for quite young people. Sugar can be found in many natural foods and is vital for energy production in your body, so that manufacturers who add sugar to their products claim they are only copying nature. Yet dentists and nutritionists warn against it; one expert has described it as 'pure, white and deadly', and another coined the term 'saccharine disease' to highlight its importance. How can one substance be so widespread and yet so bad for you?

The word sugar originally just meant sweet. In modern usage it refers to the smallest of the carbohydrates. Larger ones, like the starches in potatoes and cereals, are no longer sweet although they are constructed like long daisy-chains of sugar.

The commonest sugars in modern food are: *sucrose* from sugar cane or beet; *lactose* in milk, *fructose* in fruits and *glucose*, found chiefly in grapes, raisins, figs, plums and dates. Honey contains a mixture of fructose and glucose. *Maltose* occurs in the sprouting of grains but mostly in brewing; few people eat malt regularly.

Throughout most of history all these foods have been valued and eaten whole because of their sweetness, and no harm ever came of this. Honey was hard to find and harvest, and appetite for all the other sugars was limited by the volume of fibrous material you had to eat along with it: one average sized sugar beet, for example, would contain only about an ounce of sugar. Furthermore, this same fibrous material slows down the rate at which your digestion can release the sugars from your intestine so that your pancreas never has more than a thin trickle of sugar to cope with.

The problems started with refinement, which became affordable in the twentieth century (Chapter Five). The overall effect of refinement is to separate sweetness from its original food, so that this attractive property could be added to anything unpalatable that a food manufacturer wanted to sell. Sugar thus joined vinegar, salt and spices as the earliest food additives, but it rapidly overtook all the others and became unshakeably supreme.

Consequently, the average sugar consumption in England rose in a century from a pound a year to around two pounds (1 kilogram) per week. Forty per cent of that is pure granulated sugar and the rest is hidden in a wide variety of manufactured products, from soup mix to sweets. We have to try to cut this down. Sugar is the most highly refined substance we eat. It comes without any of the trace nutrients you need to metabolise it, that would have been present in sweet whole foods. So to burn sugar you have to steal these nutrients from your other food. But if you eat much sugar you will have little appetite left for good food! Consequently your general nutrition suffers disproportionately, especially in childhood: the scene is then set for chronic disease later in life.

What to do

1. Note all the packets you buy that mention sugar on their labels. Lots have it in the top three by quantity. Decide to stop buying these from next week. Each week make further cuts until you've painlessly got right of it all. Even then,

remember some with less than 5 per cent sugar do not list it as an ingredient, so move into fresh items instead of packets.

2. Then avoid the following intense sweeteners too: sucrose, glucose, dried or hydrogenated glucose syrup, hydrogenated high maltose glucose syrup, dextrose, fructose, invert sugar, isomalt, lactose, maltose and xylitol. Aspartame may produce a different range of problems so don't switch to that instead.

3. Choose wholemeal flour and bread, which release sugar slowly and safely. Use dried fruit to sweeten your baking. Get to like hot drinks without any sweetener at all.

4. Set your children an excellent example, even if you sneak chocolate when they're not around. Grandparents, find better ways to indulge your grandchildren than sweets, ice-cream and cake. If you 'treat' them, make it fruit.

5. If you have diabetic relatives, you or your children may be susceptible. See that you get whole wheat regularly for the chromium and manganese they contain, both vital to the health of your pancreas. A regular helping of raw carrot, and lemon juice instead of milk in tea, both have antidiabetic properties. It is wise to obtain a hair mineral analysis (call WellDesk for details – see Useful Addresses) and supplement this diet with food-state minerals in which you are deficient or borderline – GTF-chromium, zinc and manganese are particularly important. Be sure to exercise regularly to keep reasonably fit. Do not allow yourself to get appreciably overweight.

Chapter Eleven: Eating Out

Provided that your regular day-to-day routine follows the principles you have been reading about in earlier chapters, and provided you don't have any other undiagnosed complaint, you will eventually regain a normal predictable gut with no inconvenient IBS symptoms. You will then probably get away with an occasional departure from routine, without any mishap at all.

The bigger the departure, however, the chancier it is. And the more often you make exceptions, the more likely you are to get repercussions. It may seem a nuisance but you have to accept that your body, once it is used to being treated well, is less tolerant of major lapses than it seemed to be before, and throws them off more vigorously. That takes the form of symptoms for a day or two, which may even be brisker and more intrusive than you used to have before you sorted yourself out. But by the time they are over you are indeed sorted out again, back much more quickly to the stable condition it originally took you months to achieve.

These cautionary words are reason enough to take as few chances as possible. Most risks arise away from home, so let's take a look at the obstacles you face when eating out, and how to overcome them.

THE PRIVATE DINNER PARTY

You won't want to make a fuss at a friend's house – still less to set yourself up as the topic of mealtime conversation. So, if your hostess asks you in advance if you have any taboo foods you say 'No'. Your friend's party is not the time to make an issue of losing weight: your prime objective is to avoid a bout of IBS.

Arrive on time, already in a relaxed mood. That means you must not set yourself an impossible timetable in the hour beforehand, nor risk delays in traffic. Decline nibbles but accept a drink – fruit juice if you're driving, or if you prefer it. Make it long rather than short, so as not to get thirsty during the meal – but if there's a risk of that, drink plenty of water before you arrive.

When the starter is served, eat it without bread. You can choose not to take a roll in the first place, or leave on your plate any you find already there. If the starter is served on toast you face a dilemma, but your best move is simply to leave the toast uneaten, without comment except how delicious it was. Never mind any looks you may get about your manners.

When it comes to the main course, accept all the offerings on to your plate in the usual way, but eat your way slowly through most of the non-starchy vegetables first. Leave a few, to make your sequence less conspicuous. This may nevertheless provoke an attentive hostess to offer you more, which you can graciously accept or decline according to your appetite: just leave more of the second portion uneaten. Don't, for the sake of inner peace, weaken into mixing the foods on your plate – however strong the looks you get.

In due course, move on to the protein dish – still taking your time. Eat all you want of that, without any more thought of vegetables. Turn to potatoes, pasta or rice last of all, out of hunger or to mop up that delicious sauce – potatoes are more digestible, so less troublesome, than bread or rice. Once you have started on any of these starchy items, however, do not on any account return to meat.

When it comes to dessert you may have an element of choice. Your safest is cheese accompanied by a wholemeal cracker – more cracker than cheese, unless you managed to get away without any starch in the previous course. In that case you can afford more cheese, since you are still on protein.

However, considerable tact is required at this point. If your hostess can be seen to have gone to a great deal of trouble to produce an elaborate confection – even a whole string of them – then you may feel obliged to try one or more. However, these days it is so commonplace to be careful about weight that you will get away with politeness portions – tasters in small quantity. Furthermore you can savour each appreciatively and exclaim about their virtues, then leave the rest. With luck chef is dying for the excuse to finish off the serving bowls anyway, after you have gone. With a little more luck, he or she will have been to equal trouble over the cheese board, in which case you can revert to the earlier plan.

The essential challenge is to get away with as little starchy food as possible, because you will almost certainly be offered coffee and probably mints or petit fours. If you've managed to keep your starch down to a token nibble, there's nothing to be lost by going a round or two. If you've fallen for a few potatoes or crispbreads, don't indulge more than a sip of coffee, but the mints probably won't do much harm.

I haven't yet mentioned drinks within the meal. In any case avoid water, on basic principles. Wine should come in for the same treatment as bread and dessert: accept a little as politeness, taste it reflectively, praise it if you sincerely can, then leave most of it. If you do this properly there is very little risk of your even approaching the drink-drive limit by the time you depart, which makes for a happier time. If you would feel cheated on this regime, and aren't driving in any case, then request wine as your pre-prandial drink. If you get there early, as already advised, you may get lucky and be offered a second glass whilst awaiting the late-comers.

These precautions will see you safe from the digestive point of view. There is no guarantee, however, on two particular counts. One: you may get a dose of some pesticide you have been diligently avoiding for months, in which case you can flush it out with a few days on garlic oil (see Chapter Ten, Cleansing Diet).

And two, you may still come under interrogation from your hostess, or even another guest, despite your attempt to keep a low profile. You will have to decide on the spot, according to the sincerity or otherwise of the line of questioning. You can try to parry with something like 'Yes, it is strange, isn't it? I always eat this way – I find it more comfortable'. That should put off any suspicion that you dislike what's on offer, but it won't deflect genuine curiosity. I wouldn't be led into a discussion of bowels at the dinner table, but I suppose you could blame it all on a doctor's theory you're trying out, then smartly turn the tables on your inquisitor and change the subject. A genuine seeker after truth will take the hint, and have a quiet word with you over coffee.

RESTAURANTS

At a private party you usually get to see what's on offer before you're served. The problem at a restaurant is that the menu may not betray much about what you'll be getting. In some fast food establishments the meals arrive partly prepared out of house, so the waiters can't add much of value to what the menu says. Therefore, only go where your meal is likely to be cooked for you, freshly and individually. That way you can expect your preferences to carry some weight. The food may even be at least as good as you would prepare yourselves at home. The cost will be a little more, but to eat out well more seldom is the wiser habit.

Take your time over the menu, whilst enjoying a glass of water followed by another of fresh juice This may raise the waiter's eyebrows but won't unsettle your companions. If the menu is unintelligible, get the waiter to explain key items for you before you order.

It makes sense to choose a fresh salad or melon to begin with. Vegetable soup should go down well. Avoid pate, because it's very inelegant to eat it without toast and you have blown your course sequence right out of the water. My usual choice is avocado salad.

The main course these days is usually less of a problem than it was, because vegetables are likely to be separate. I generally go for fish if it's available but may indulge in something else, like venison or Scottish beef that we would never have at home. Try to avoid pasta, pizza or rice with a meaty sauce already on it, which makes separation virtually impossible. Neither rice nor pasta is anywhere near as digestible as potato, and a distinct gap between meat and these starches is very wise.

Strangely enough, the vegetarian options available in restaurants are often the least digestible dishes on the menu. They usually combine pastry, rice or pasta indiscriminately with eggs, cheese or beans and are often not very imaginative. Generally speaking, you will do better to have a generous selection of vegetables, and an omelette if you are not vegan.

Otherwise much the same applies as in a private meal. Decline the roll, even with soup. Leave potatoes, rice and pasta alone if you fancy a bash at the dessert trolley.

ETHNIC CUISINE

I very much like French, Middle Eastern, Indian and Chinese food and it is possible to arrange any of these in a perfectly digestible order. In the Orient you would be served rice only at the end of a meal, not with it. Even in Europe the Chinese use their chopsticks to pick up morsels from the richer dishes and eat them off the top of their bowls of rice, leaving that until last. We eat our Indian food in just the same way, and have in both cases ordered progressively less rice over the years. We avoid Biryiani-style dishes since the rice is combined in them, not served separately.

Thai, Indian and Indonesian food can contain very hot spices. It would be wise to avoid these, and choose milder dishes. Cuisine from northern India is generally mild, getting progressively hotter as you move south. Restaurants vary, however, and you will need to check with the waiter what the menu means by 'medium'.

The chief problem arises with Italian food. I had hoped I would find that the Italians, like the Chinese, arrange things differently at home; but it appears not. A dish of pasta with a sauce is likely to be served somewhere in the middle of the main meal, second or third of perhaps five courses. Pizza presents even more difficult problems. What point is there in ordering one, only to eat the topping off before dealing with the bread base? I have to confess this has me foxed, and in general I don't choose to eat either of these flagship items in Italian restaurants. But we are off to Italy this summer to find out whether there is something I have missed. If things get desperate, we can always retreat into France.

CODA

Useful Addresses

This is an alphabetical index of all the self-help agencies and sources of professional assistance that have been mentioned throughout this book, and a few that haven't.

Biodynamic
See Organic

Colitis and Crohn's Disease, National Association
This group, some 20,000 strong, provides support and information for sufferers of all forms of bowel disorder. Annual membership is inexpensive and includes free copies of many useful publications. Tel. 01727 844296 (a very busy line); or contact www.nacc.org.uk, or write to NACC, 4 Beaumont House, Sutton Road, St Albans, Herts AL1 5HH.

Colonic Therapist
For a fully trained and reliable practitioner contact The Association and Register of Colon Therapists. Tel: 01442 827687; or write to: 16 Drummond Ride, Tring, Hertfordshire HP23 5DE. The website www.colonic-association.com is independent of them.

Cytoplan Ltd
A company that supplies equipment and food-state supplements largely to health professionals, they can also be approached for advice and supplies by members of the public. Their aloe vera gel 10:1 concentrate is recommended. They supply and advise on the use of enema equipment. Tel: helpline 01507 608882; order line 01684 310099; or write to Cytoplan Ltd, 8 Hanley Workshops, Hanley Road, Hanley Swan, Worcs WR8 0DX.

Food-state™
Food-state™ nutrients are manufactured in the USA by Grow Company Inc, 195 Kenneth Street, PO Box 838, Hackensack, NJ 07601. Tel. 201 342 2007.

Good HealthKeeping
This is a health service for subscribers, who pay £11 per family or household per quarter-year (first six months £30). Its object is to help you live your life to the full, with minimal reliance on doctors or medicines. Subscribers have access to a professionally staffed call-centre, trained and supervised personally by Dr Mansfield, from 9–6 on weekdays and 9–12 on Saturday (except Bank Holidays). They get supplies by post at little over cost price. An extensive list of leaflets, a password-protected website a fluoride laboratory service and a health-score questionnaire are available to them free of further charge. There is a topical monthly newsletter.

Tel. 08707 HEALTH (432584); or write to Good HealthKeeping, PO Box 6, Louth, LN11 8XL.

Henry Doubleday Research Association
The premier source for practical advice on and supplies for organic gardening, from windowbox to wide open acres. They have a membership of over 30,000 and their demonstration gardens at Ryton and Yalding (Kent) are well worth visiting for useful ideas. Tel. 024 7630 3517; or write to: HDRA, Ryton Organic Gardens, Coventry CV8 3LG; or e-mail enquiry@ hdra.org.uk.

Herbs
Hambleden Herbs are a reputable organic herb farm with an extensive catalogue and efficient mail order service. Tel. 018 2340 1205; or write to: Court Farm, Milverton, Somerset TA4 1NE.

Homoeopathy
This is the safest way to get good symptomatic relief of your gut symptoms whilst solving the underlying problems in the long term. Several High Street chemists and health shops now stock a range of low-potency self-help remedies, and can give basic

advice or literature to guide your choice. If you cannot find one locally, contact Weleda (UK) Ltd. Tel. 011 5944 8200; or write to: Heanor Road, Ilkeston, Derbyshire DE7 8DR. They have several very useful publications and expert staff who can dispense for you by post directly if necessary.

You may need specific help to deal with miasms, from a Psionic Medical Practitioner (below).

Naturopath

This term is attributed to Benedict Lust, an American pioneer of natural therapy. It refers to a healing practitioner who relies on methods available in nature, such as diet, water, breathing, massage and herbal remedies. Several training and registration bodies exist across the world, but the discipline has not yet achieved in Britain the professional standing it enjoys in the USA. Contact the General Council and Register of Naturopaths. Tel. 014 5884 0072; or write to: Goswell House, 2 Goswell Road, Street, Somerset BA16 0JG for a qualified naturopath near you.

Organic food

This term covers food grown without the use of artificial fertilisers or crop protection chemicals, which requires the use of composted biological matter as fertilizer. It derives from the work of agricultural pioneers such as Sir Albert Howard and Lady Eve Balfour, upon which the work of The Soil Association Ltd was built. This has become the foremost standard-bearer and regulator of organic agriculture in Britain. Tel. 011 7926 0661, or write to Bristol House, 40–56 Victoria Street, Bristol BS1 6BY, or e-mail info@soilassociation. org, website www.soil association.org.

Soil Association
Symbol of Organic Quality

The Biodynamic Agriculture Association take their commitment to natural farming a step further by requiring that their crops are part of a whole farming ecosystem. Their work springs from the insights of Rudolph Steiner and they regulate the Demeter quality mark, which is not so well known or widely available in Britain as the Soil Association symbol. Further details may be had from The Biodynamic Agricultural Association. Tel/Fax. 014 5375 8501, or write to: The Painswick Inn Project, Gloucester Street, Stroud, Glos GL5 1QG or e-mail: bdaa@biodynamic.freeserve.co.uk; website: www.anth.org.uk/biodynamic.

The US biodynamic address is Demeter Association Inc, Britt Road, Aurora, NY 13026. Tel. 315 364 5617; fax. 315 364 5224; website www.demeter-usa.org.

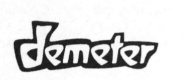 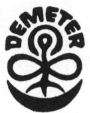

Psionic Medicine

This is a specialised form of homoeopathy in which removal of miasms (Chapter Four) is emphasised. Practitioners are medically qualified and are able to analyse a sample of blood or hair sent by post, with a covering letter. Contact Dr Pam Tatham, Secretary, Institute of Psionic Medicine, 79 Hallgarth Street, Durham DH1 3AY.

Water purifiers

The best water for drinking is virtually pure, with only very low levels of minerals dissolved in it. All the additives from water processing are undesirable. There are only two ways to remove them all – distillation and reverse osmosis. I recommend reverse osmosis because the ongoing costs are lower and the water is not overpurified. The apparatus is plumbed into your kitchen sink and a separate tap provided. It occupies about a third of the space of one standard under-sink kitchen cupboard. Kits for self-installation are available from Good HealthKeeping (see above) for around £230 all inclusive. Maintenance is recommended every two to four years, depending on the condition of your mains water supply, and costs at most about £25 per year.

Websites

www.ibsgroup.org is the most informative, least commercial site at the time of writing.

www.bsg.org.uk is the British Society of Gastro-enterologists, or gut specialist doctors, for those with a professional or technical interest. It is not confined to IBS, however.

www.ibs-register.co.uk deals with hypnotherapy as a means of improving IBS, which I have not otherwise touched on in this book.

Solvay Pharmaceuticals have a site dealing with their bowel-related products at www.solvay-ibs.com, but it carries general information too.

WellDesk

This is a service for non-members, provided by Good Health-Keeping (see above). There is a free website – www.welldesk. com – and a premium rate call centre on 0906 802 0 803. You will be charged 60p per minute but will not waste any time talking to intermediaries – your call is answered by a professional health adviser, under the direct supervision of a doctor experienced in health and natural medicines. The conversation will be limited to 15 minutes on any one occasion. You should seek your GP's advice as well.

Bibliography

The following is a consolidated list of books and scientific papers referred to in the text, together with some additional titles of background interest to the topic of this book.

AM. J. MED. (1999). 107, Supplement 8 November.
—— (2000). A systematic review of water fluoridation. NHS Centre for Reviews and Dissemination, University of York, Report 18.
BARBARA, L. *et al.* (1991). Pathogenesis of irritable bowel syndrome. *Ital. J. Gastroenterol.* 23, Suppl. 1. 36–38.
BARNES, B.O. (1976). *Solved: The Riddle of Heart Attacks.* Fort Collins, Colorado: Robinson Press.
BIRCHER-BENNER, M. (1959). *The Prevention of Incurable Disease.* London: James Clark, 2nd Edition.
CAMILLERI, M. & PRATHER, C.M. (1992). The irritable bowel syndrome: mechanisms and a practical approach to management. *Annals of Internal Medicine.* 116, I001–8.
CHOUDHARY, N.A. & TRUELOVE, S.C. (1962). The irritable colon syndrome. A study of the clinical features, predisposing causes and prognosis in 130 cases. *Q.J. Med.* 31, 307–322.
CLEAVE, T.L. (1974). *The Saccharine Disease,* Bristol: Wright.
—— (1990). Dietary fibre, food intolerance and irritable bowel syndrome. *Nutritional Reviews.* 48, 343–6.
EHRET, A. (1994). *The Mucusless Diet Healing System,* Ehret Literature Publ. Co., Inc., Ardsley, N.Y. 10502–2613 USA.
GRANT, D. & JOICE, J. (1984). *Food Combining for Health.* London: Thorsons.
HABGOOD, J. (1997) *The Hay Diet Made Easy,* London: Souvenir Press.
HAHNEMANN, SAMUEL (1810). *The Organon of the Rational System of Medicine.* Currently 1992; London: Victor Gollancz.

HAY, W.J. (1934). *Health via Food*, London: Harrap.

HUGILL, J.A.C. (1949). Sugar. London: Coomes.

KNEIPP, S. (1891). *My Water Cure*. London: Blackwood.

LANE, W.A. (1935). *The New Health Guide*. London: Bles.

MCCARRISON, R. (1921). *Studies in Deficiency Disease*. London: Hodder & Stoughton.

MANNING, A.P. *et al.* (1978). Towards positive diagnosis of the irritable bowel. *BMJ*. 2, 653–4.

MANSFIELD, P. & MONRO, J. (1987). *Chemical Children*. London: Century. (out of print but available from Good HealthKeeping)

MONTIGNAC, M. (1991). *Eat Yourself Slim*. UK: Artulen.

OLDFIELD, H. & COGHILL, R. (1988). *The Dark Side of the Brain*. Shaftesbury: Element Books.

PICTON, L.J. (1946). *Thoughts on Feeding*. London: Faber & Faber.

PIRSIG, ROBERT (1974). *Zen and the Art of Motorcycle Maintenance*. London: Bodley Head.

POTTENGER, F.M. (1983). *Pottenger's Cats*. Price-Pottenger.

PRICE, W.A. (1970). *Nutrition and Physical Degeneration*. Price-Pottenger Foundation.

REYNER, J.M. (2001). *Psionic Medicine*. London: CW Daniel.

SAXTON BURR, HAROLD (1972). *Blueprint for immortality*. London: Neville Spearman.

SHELDRAKE, RUPERT (1988). *The Presence of the Past*. London: Harper Collins.

SMITH, CYRIL & BEST, SIMON (1989). *Electromagnetic Man*. London: Dent.

SMOUT, A. *et al.* (2000). Potential pitfalls in the differential diagnosis of irritable bowel syndrome. *Digestion*. 61, 247–56.

STEINER, RUDOLPH (1981). *Health and Illness*. Volume 1, Anthroposophic Press. (Among many other titles)

WAERLAND, A. (1934). *In the Cauldron of Disease*. London: Nutt (Berry).

WALDBOTT, G.L. (1978). *Fluoridation, The Great Dilemma*. Lawrence Kansas: Coronade Press.

WILLIAMSON, GEORGE S. & PEARSE, I.H. (1980). *Science, Synthesis and Sanity*, Scottish Academic Press.

Index

NB – no foods are listed here – look for them in Chapter Nine. Food Families (Latin names) appear only in Chapter Ten. Information sources are listed in Useful Addresses. Authors are listed in the Bibliography.

Acidophilus   27, **85–86**, 130
Aluminium   59, **64**, 92, 142
Antrum   **31–32,** 75, 79, 113
Appendicitis   62, 64, **91–94**, 125, 126
Appendix   85, 90–91
Assimilation   **72**, 80
Béchamp   17
Beeton   **49**
Bio-technology   60
Bowel   4–9, 25–27, 29, 66, 76, **84–101**
Cadmium   58, 64
Caecum   61, **84–86**
Calcium   108, 143
Candida albicans   **87–89**
Cardia   31
Cellulose   **26–27**, 83–86, 119, 133
Chromosome   39
Codeine   62, 98
Coeliac Disease   5–8
Colon   5, 17, **90**, **94–95**, 173
Constipation   **92–94**
Crohn's Disease   5, **7–8**, 29, 173
Digestion   20, 27, 32, **74–79**, 84, 97, **106–121**
Digestive Leucocytosis   81, 110
Diverticula(r Disease)   7, 95
Diverticulitis   7, 95
Diverticulosis   7, 95
Ectoderm   71
Enzyme   30, 50, 78, 112, 114
E coli   **86–87**, 91
E number   58–60
Endoderm   71
Escherichia coli   **86–87**, 91
Fluoride   65–66
Fundus   31–32, 79, 113

Gastro-colic Reflex   98. See also 'The Cauldron of Disease' on p. 84
Gene   6–8, 22, 31, 39–40, **60–61**, 81
Distillation, of water   108, 176
DNA   13
Gut   4
Hardness, of water   108
Health   15–20, **174**
Heredity   6, **39–41**
Indigestion   3–4, 7
Inflammatory Bowel Disease   5, 62, 81, 110
Intestine   4
Lead   64
Leibig   51
Leucocytosis   81, 110
Mackeith   57
McLaren-Howard   66
Magnesium   108
Mercury   64
Miasm   42
NPK   51
Patent   14
Pesticide   6, 54, 62–64, 82, 92
Pholcodeine   62, 98
Piles   95
Pylorus   31–32, 79
Reverse Osmosis   65, **108**, 176
Scalar   40
'Soul'   39–45
Starch   26, **30**
Stomach   4, 28, **31–32**
Syndrome   5
Tea   66, **106, 128**
Thrush   **87–89**
Truss   88
Ulcerative Colitis   7–8